Ho…
Treat

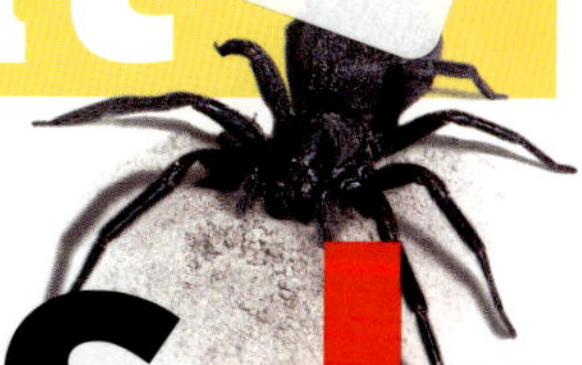

Bites + Stings

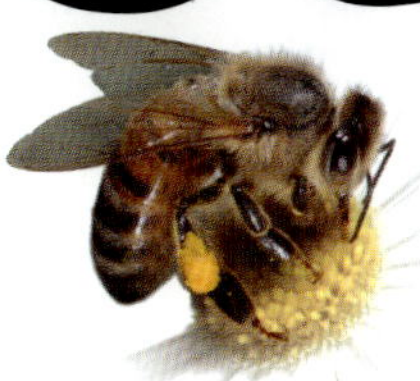

Gerry and Marlene Swan

ACKNOWLEDGEMENTS

Thanks to our colleagues and friends who have provided information and images for this book, and the CSIRO for allowing us to photograph specimens of the Whiplash Rove Beetle. Thanks also to our family for acting as models and coming up with sources of information and images—in particular Jodi for finding hard-to-get information and confirming first-aid techniques, and Geoff for photography and sourcing other photographs.

First published in Australia in 2006 by
Reed New Holland
an imprint of New Holland Publishers (Australia) Pty Ltd
Sydney • Auckland • London • Cape Town
14 Aquatic Drive Frenchs Forest NSW 2086 Australia
218 Lake Road Northcote Auckland New Zealand
86 Edgware Road London W2 2EA United Kingdom
80 McKenzie Street Cape Town 8001 South Africa

National Library of Australia
Cataloguing-in-Publication Data:

Swan, Gerry.
How to treat bites and stings.

Includes index.
ISBN 1 877069 36 1.

1. Bites and stings - Treatment - Australia.
2. Venom - Physiological effect - Australia.
3. Poisonous animals - Venom - Toxicology - Australia.
4. First aid in illness and injury. I. Swan, Marlene.
II. Title.

615.9420994

Publisher: Martin Ford
Project Editor: Yani Silvana
Designer: Norman Baptista, Nota Bene Design
Cover Design: Greg Lamont
Deep etched images: Hypermouse
Production: Linda Bottari
Printer: Tien Wah Press, Malaysia

CONTENTS

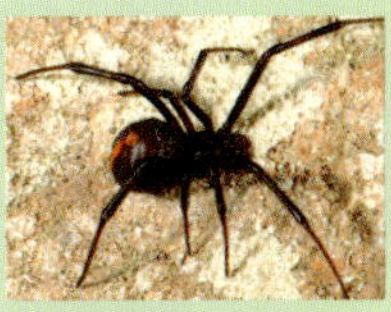

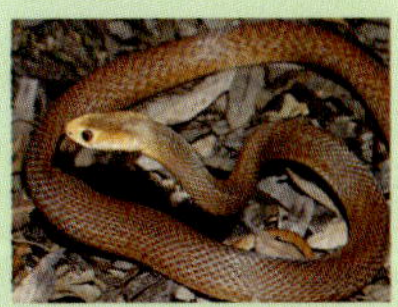

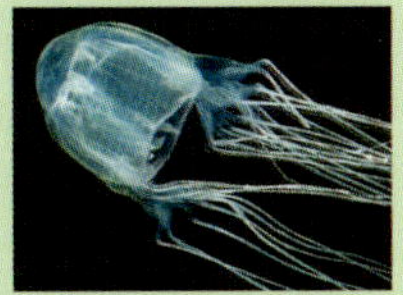

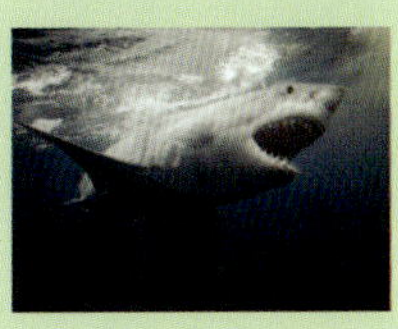

INTRODUCTION

AUSTRALIA IS full of creatures that bite and sting. Even some plants sting or are poisonous. Some are dangerous and life threatening, others are just a damn nuisance. This book covers both the very dangerous and the simply annoying.

Most people don't even know what is dangerous and what is not. 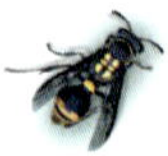 Information on symptoms and first aid is often buried in reams of other text within books or on the Internet and is not readily accessible in an emergency. And to top it off, the book won't stay open on the page you want because of the binding (not a problem with this book).

We have not covered every possible source of a bite or sting—that would run to many hundreds of pages. But we have included those that you are most likely to encounter at home, at the beach or in the country. For completeness some of the more spectacular bites, such as crocodiles and sharks, have been included. Poisonous plants and fungi are mentioned but not comprehensively covered.

In writing this book it became apparent how important it is that individuals learn what to do in an emergency. At least one person in a family should complete a recognised first-aid course. Families should have a comprehensive first-aid kit in the house and in the car—not just the usual bandaids, small bandages and safety pins, but bandages suitable for pressure bandaging, as well as local anaesthetic and other medications, and resuscitation masks (see page 9 for suggested first-aid kit).

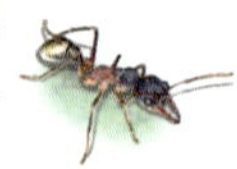

HOW TO USE THIS BOOK

THIS BOOK is intended as a practical reference book to help you identify what has caused a particular bite or sting and what first aid to apply. The creatures or plants are listed in alphabetical order by common name; where more than one common name is in use, all are included in the index at the back of the book.

At the beginning of each account, a star rating ranging from one to four indicates the degree of danger associated with a bite or sting from the species described.

★	Annoying, temporary discomfort. Not regarded as dangerous.
★★	Some discomfort. Not dangerous unless the victim has an allergy.
★★★	Potentially dangerous. Capable of causing marked local symptoms. Always seek medical aid.
★★★★	Extremely dangerous. Capable of causing death. Always seek medical aid.

Each entry opens with a brief description of the creature, including its approximate length. Read this in conjunction with the photographs to assist identification. However, it is not always possible to give detailed descriptions. For example, there are some 600 known species of sea urchin, of which about 80 are dangerous to people. By including sea urchins in this book we are letting readers know that some can cause problems, and that all should be left alone. This applies to most creatures, whether they are snakes, spiders, caterpillars or jellyfish.

Within the description is an indication of the regions in which the organism may occur. This does not mean that it is found everywhere within that area. Many animals have quite specific habitat requirements and the distribution of a species is unlikely to be continuous throughout its known range. Maps giving distribution are also given.

PHOTOGRAPHS or illustrations showing the organism in question accompany the text. However, there may be wide colour variation, or many species may be involved, so we can only provide a few typical examples.

SYMPTOMS described are those that usually occur, but a victim may not experience all or any of these.

FIRST-AID TECHNIQUES given are simple and can be applied by anyone attempting to assist the victim. However, in many cases you will also need to call for qualified medical assistance.

EMERGENCY PHONE NUMBERS

Poisons Information Centre:
13 11 26 from anywhere in Australia

The Poisons Information Centre gives advice on bites and stings, any time, from anywhere in Australia.

Australian Venom Research Unit
24-hour advisory line: 03 8344 7753

Ambulance: (or dial 000)

Hospital:

Doctor:

24-hour chemist:

PREVENTION

PREVENTING A bite or sting is better than having to treat one. While many bites and stings are merely a nuisance, some are life threatening—some jellyfish (also known as sea jellies), sharks, some spiders and snakes, to name a few.

More individuals and families are engaging in recreational activities in marine environments, outback regions, or in national parks and reserves, where they may encounter potentially harmful creatures and plants. But even people who lead an essentially suburban existence should be aware of the harmful creatures that occur in their area, be able to identify them, and minimise contact.

Common sense is the best prevention against bites and stings:

- If it is something you are unfamiliar with, leave it and its home (nest, burrow etc.) alone.
- Always wear appropriate clothing and footwear for the occasion. For example: wear gloves when cleaning up in the garden or exploring rock pools or reefs; wear closed shoes when walking in the bush, in the garden or on reefs, or when wading in muddy water; wear long trousers when walking in areas prone to leeches or to such plants as stinging nettles.
- Don't swim in muddy waters, or in areas where there has been a recent shark attack, or near seal colonies. Use netted areas when possible.
- Don't spearfish.
- Pay attention to any warning notices.
- Do not wade, swim or fish in tropical waterways, and do not camp next to them.
- Don't swim in the ocean in jellyfish-prone climates.
- Wild animals are just that—wild. They are not pets or companion animals, and their response to being handled or approached is unpredictable. Teach your children not to handle animals with which they are unfamiliar. Teasing or tormenting any animal is completely unjustifiable.
- Avoid areas where biting and stinging insects proliferate.

- Screen windows and doors at home and discourage birds from roosting on window ledges or in the roof.
- Don't leave clothes lying on the floor overnight (spiders).
- Check inside shoes and gloves before putting them on, particularly if they are stored outside (gumboots, gardening gloves).
- Check yourself and children for ticks if you've been in the bush or tick-prone areas.
- Use a good insect repellent.

First-Aid Kit

St John Ambulance Australia and The Australian Red Cross have comprehensive first-aid kits for the home and the car.

A kit should contain:

- A range of bandages to bind dressings in place. These should include triangular bandages for use as slings and two 10–20cm crepe bandages for pressure immobilisation.
- A range of dressing pads.
- Gauze swabs and alcohol swabs.
- A roll of adhesive tape.
- Bandaids.
- Disposable gloves and towels.
- Thermo blanket.
- Stainless steel scissors.
- Stainless steel tweezers.
- Safety pins.
- Reusable ice pack.
- Resuscitation mouth mask.
- First-aid manual.
- Notepad and pencil.
- Antiseptic cream.
- Local anaesthetic preparation such as Stingose™.
- Analgesics.

THIS BOOK provides general first aid for common bites and stings. Many are not dangerous—just irritating or painful. Others are extremely dangerous.

We have included basic life-support techniques, although these would rarely be required, but we strongly recommend that readers undergo formal first-aid training so that they know what to do in case of an accident or emergency. Be alert to possible dangers at the scene and always ensure your own safety.

Recovery Position

Place an unconscious person in the recovery position while you clear their airway, and to maintain them in a stable position.

- Kneel beside victim.
- Position victim on back and straighten limbs.
- Lift nearer leg so it is fully bent.
- Place nearer arm across chest.
- Place further arm at right angles to body.
- Roll victim away from you onto side, with leg at right angles and knee touching the ground.
- If necessary, check that airway is open and clear.

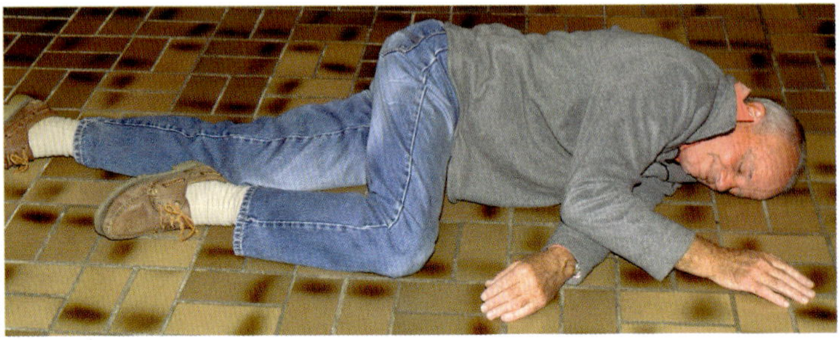

GEOFF SWAN

Recovery position

Expired Air Resuscitation (EAR)

When someone stops breathing the aim is to prevent irreversible damage or death by supplying oxygen to the vital organs until normal breathing recommences or expert medical aid can take over.

- Handle unconscious victims carefully to avoid neck and spinal injuries.
- Make sure that airway is open. Place victim in the recovery position (see page 10) and open their mouth to allow drainage of vomit or secretions. Clear any solids with your fingers.
- Roll victim onto back and tilt head backwards by placing the palm of your hand on top of victim's forehead and applying firm pressure. With your other hand lift victim's jaw forward and open the mouth.
- Kneel beside victim's head, close victim's nostrils with your thumb and forefinger, and place your other hand gently on the chin to keep mouth open without placing pressure on the soft tissues of the neck.

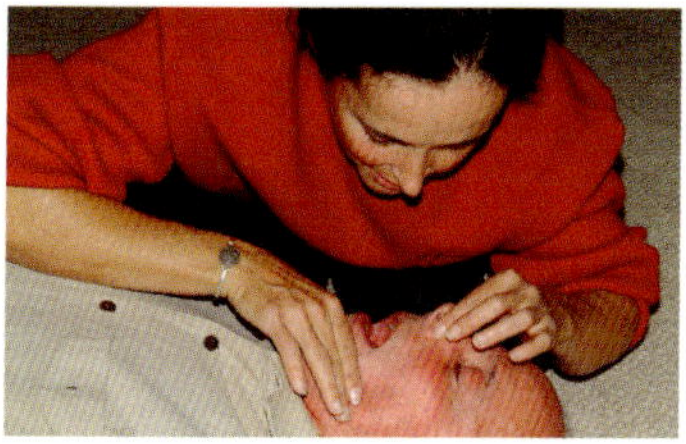

GEOFF SWAN

Resuscitating

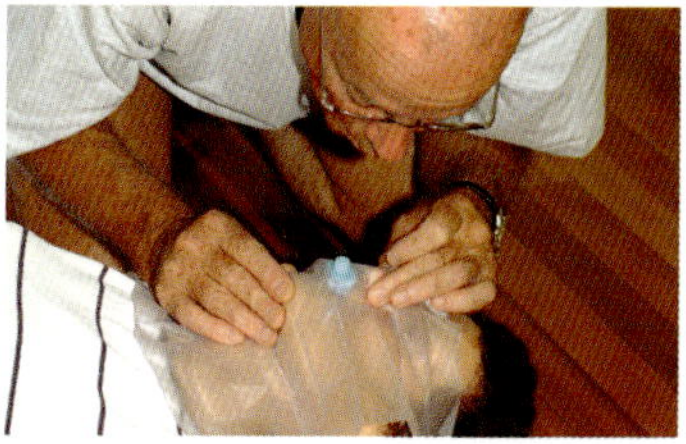

GEOFF SWAN

Using a resuscitation mask

- Your first-aid kit should contain a resusciation mask. Use it to avoid mouth-to-mouth contact. Take a deep breath, place your mouth over victim's mouth, making an airtight seal, and breath into victim's mouth. At the same time turn your head to see that the chest rises. If it does not, the airway is not clear and you must recheck the mouth and throat.

- Remove your mouth from victim's and watch for victim's chest to fall.
- Repeat this rapidly for five breaths, then check pulse (see box).
- If there is no pulse, commence cardiopulmonary resuscitation (CPR) immediately (see below).
- If pulse is present, continue resuscitation at the rate of one breath every five seconds.
- Recheck for breathing and pulse after one minute, then at two-minute intervals.
- If victim recommences breathing, turn them to the recovery position.

CHILDREN For babies and young children just support the jaw (don't tilt the head backwards), put your mouth over the child's nose and mouth and breathe gently and shallowly. Gently breathe enough air into the child's lungs to make the chest rise lightly.

Checking for a Pulse

If the heart has stopped there will be no pulse at the wrist or neck.

To check for a pulse at the wrist, place your first two fingers (not the thumb) firmly across the wrist on the palm side. The artery runs down the wrist at about the ball of the thumb, and you will feel a pulse (if there is one) at the wrist below this point.

To check for a pulse at the neck, place two fingers (not thumb) in the groove on one side of the windpipe.

Cardiopulmonary Resuscitation (CPR)

Use this technique when you can't find a pulse and the victim has stopped breathing.

- Lay victim on a firm, level surface, not a bed; make sure the head is not higher than the body.

- Position yourself beside victim's chest.
- Place a finger at the point where the lowest ribs meet in the centre of the chest.
- Place a finger in the groove between the collarbones, immediately below the throat.
- Find the half-way point between these two locations and place the heel of one hand on this spot. Your fingers should be slightly raised pointing across the chest.
- Place your other hand on top of the first, with the fingers between the fingers of the first hand.
- With arms straight and shoulders above the victim, use your body weight to depress the breastbone 4–5cm. Apply 15 compressions in 10 seconds, followed by two breaths in five seconds.
- Complete four of these cycles each minute. Check for pulse and breathing after one minute, then at two-minute intervals.
- If pulse returns, continue with EAR until breathing returns.

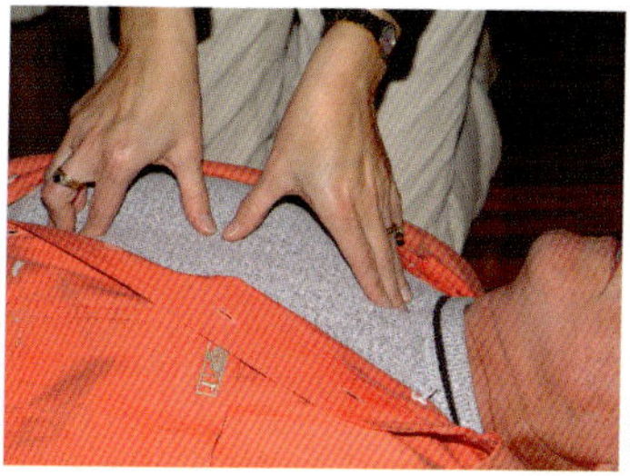

GEOFF SWAN

Locating the spot

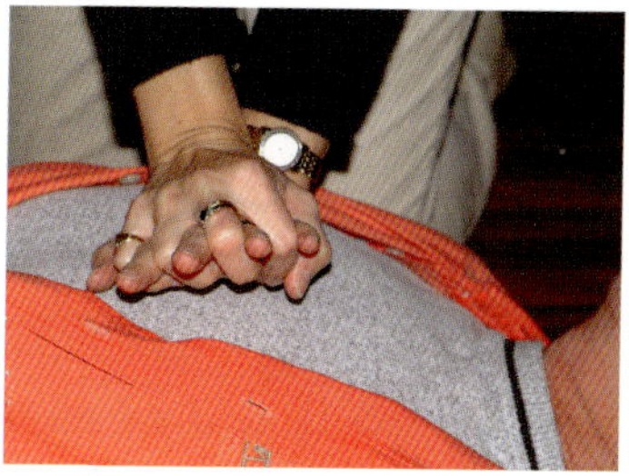

GEOFF SWAN

Hands on breastbone

CHILDREN For a child use one hand and depress the breastbone 2–3cm. For an infant use two fingers and depress 1–2cm. Complete six cycles each minute.

Bleeding

Some bites may be associated with significant blood loss and your priority is to stop the bleeding.

- Apply direct pressure to the wound by firmly placing a cloth or pad onto the site. If you have no cloth or pad, ask the victim to apply direct pressure with their hand, or as a last resort use your own hand.
- If possible, elevate the injured area to slow the flow of blood.
- Put a clean dressing over the wound. Place a thick cloth pad that is wider than the wound on top. Bandage firmly. Do not remove when bleeding has decreased or stopped. If bleeding continues, reposition the pad and re-bandage.
- Direct pressure may be unsuccessful when bleeding is severe. You will need to apply pressure to a pressure point between the wound and the heart (see diagram). You will know you have found the right spot when the bleeding stops. When the bleeding is controlled reapply the direct pressure as set out above and release pressure from the pressure point.
- If the above methods have not stopped the bleeding, you may need to use a constrictive bandage.
- Bind a wide (19cm or more) bandage or cloth strip firmly around the limb above the wound site. Tie securely and record the time the bandage was applied.
- Leave in place until the bleeding is controlled and you can't feel a pulse below the bandage.
- After 30 minutes untie the bandage and check if the bleeding recommences. If it does not, remove the constrictive bandage. If it does, reapply direct pressure. If this fails reapply the

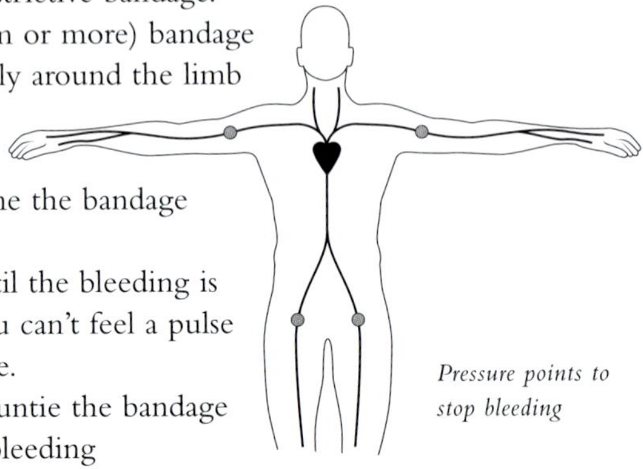

Pressure points to stop bleeding

constrictive bandage. Record the time it was reapplied and check again after 30 minutes. (Leaving the bandage on for too long can lead to tissue death from lack of blood.)

Pressure-immobilisation Technique

Use this technique for snake bite, funnel-web spider bite, blue-ringed octopus bite, box jellyfish sting or cone shell sting.

- Wrap a broad bandage firmly around the bite but not tight enough to restrict blood flow. If you don't have a bandage tear clothing or other material into strips.
- Start bandaging at the bite and continue down to the fingers or toes then go back up the limb to cover as much as possible. Try to restrict any movement of the limb while doing this, to prevent further circulation of a suspected toxin.
- Do not remove clothing—to save time, bandage over any clothing.

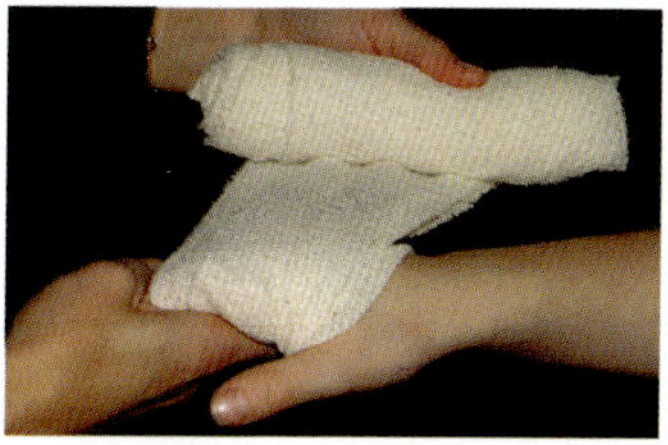
GEOFF SWAN

Start bandaging at the bite

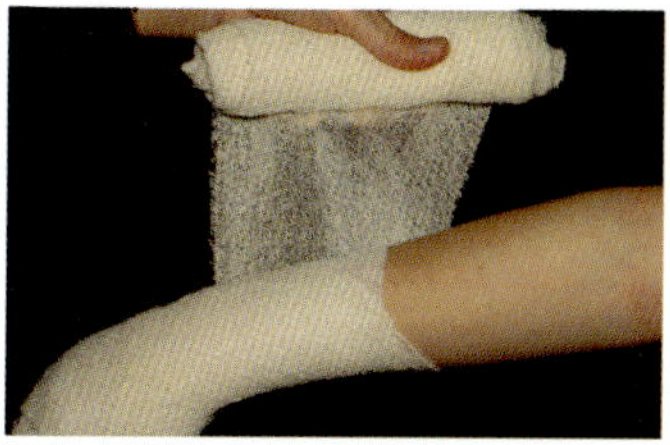
GEOFF SWAN

Continue bandaging up the limb

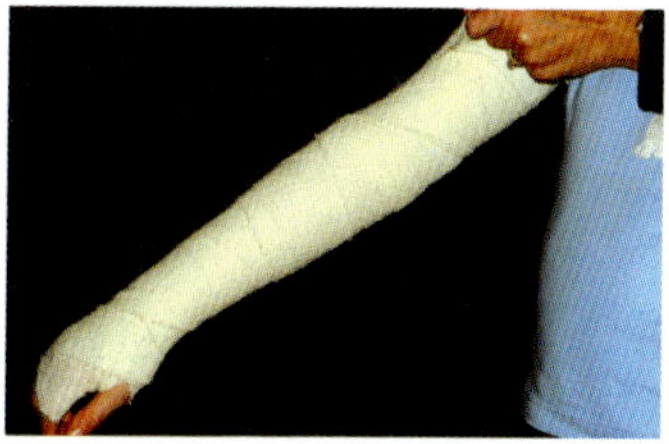
GEOFF SWAN

Bandage the whole limb

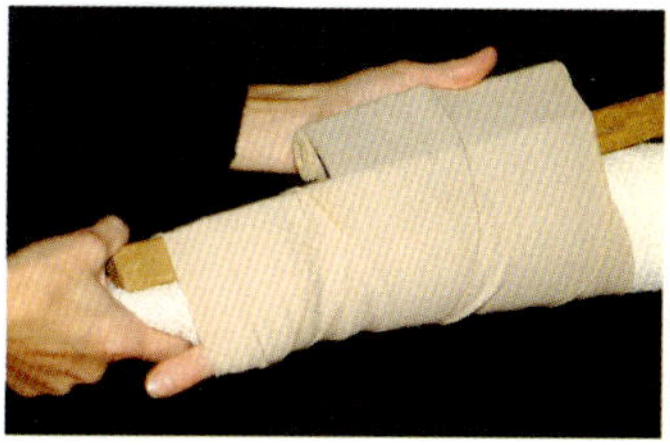
GEOFF SWAN

Fix a splint to the limb

- Fix a splint to the limb so that it cannot be moved. You may have to improvise a splint from wood, branches, rolled up newspapers or clothing. It is important to immobilise the limb to prevent muscle movement that would circulate the venom.
- It is helpful to mark the position of the bite on the bandaged limb with a pen or pencil. If the hospital needs to take a swab of the bite, the bandage can be cut at that place rather than being removed.
- Keep the victim immobile and calm. Bring transport to the victim if at all possible.
- Fortunately, bites to the face or trunk are uncommon. In such a case it may be impossible to apply a bandage. If possible hold a pad of cloth firmly against the bite and seek medical attention.

Shock

Symptoms of shock include faintness or dizziness, nausea, weak and rapid pulse, pale face, cool skin and rapid breathing.

- Lie victim down and reassure.
- Manage any bite or sting.
- Raise victim's legs above the level of their heart.
- Loosen any tight clothing and maintain body warmth.
- Check breathing and pulse.
- Put victim in the recovery position if they have breathing difficulties, are likely to vomit or become unconscious.
- Seek medical aid.

Heat Treatment

The first-aid treatment for many fish stings involves immersing or applying hot water to the site of the wound. The water should be hot but not so hot as to scald. Test the water yourself to make sure it is not too hot. Often the victim will have numbness around the wound or very severe pain and may not realise that scalding is occurring. Be particularly careful when using this treatment on children or people with sensitive skin.

If the wound cannot be immersed, apply a hot pack.

You might have to improvise and use an alternative source of heat such as hot sand or rocks, or a hot drink from a thermos.

Allergic Reaction

An allergic reaction can be caused by a substance entering the body as the result of a sting, bite, contact or inhalation. Symptoms include: redness, swelling of the skin, itching, raised rash, nausea, vomiting, swelling of the throat, wheezing, coughing, rapid, irregular pulse, dizziness or unconsciousness.

- Check breathing and pulse.
- Send for medical assistance.
- Check if victim has any medication for allergies and if so, use it.
- If victim is conscious, set them up in a comfortable position and reassure.
- If victim is unconscious, check breathing and pulse and commence EAR or CPR if necessary.

ANTS

ALL AUSTRALIAN ants bite or sting, though only a few are really painful. Ants live in large colonies that they defend fiercely, so avoid them whenever possible. Be especially wary of the following species.

BULLDOG ANT ★★

(Bullant, Jumper Ant, Bulljoe, Inchmen, Jack-jumper, Sergeant Ant)

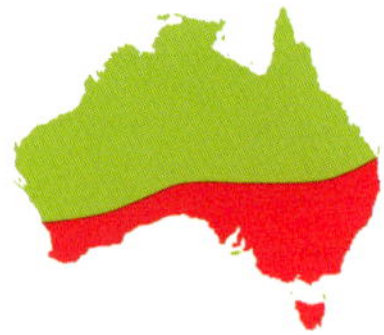

2–3 cm long. Large pincer-like jaws to hold on while injecting venom through a stinger on the tail. The stinger is only visible when in use. They vary in colour from black to dark red–brown to almost yellow. Widespread. Bushland. Some species becoming more common in the suburbs.

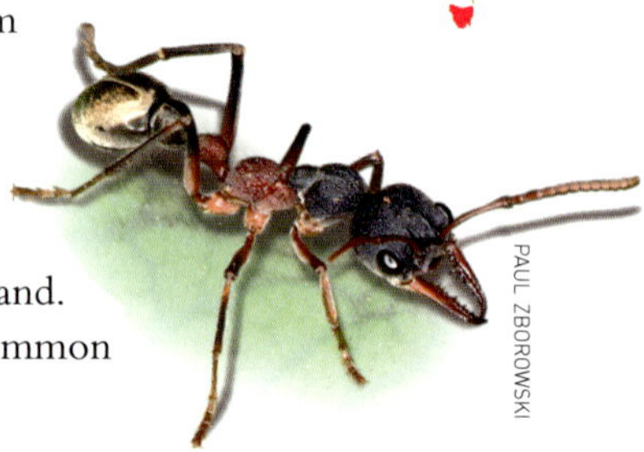

PAUL ZBOROWSKI

Symptoms

Sharp, intense pain and swelling. Pain usually abates after about half an hour, leaving a small red swelling that disappears in a few days. Rarely serious but occasionally an allergic reaction may result.

First Aid

- Move victim away from ants and remove ants from their body.
- Apply ice pack/cold compress or calamine lotion.
- If symptoms persist, seek medical aid.

RED FIRE ANT ★★

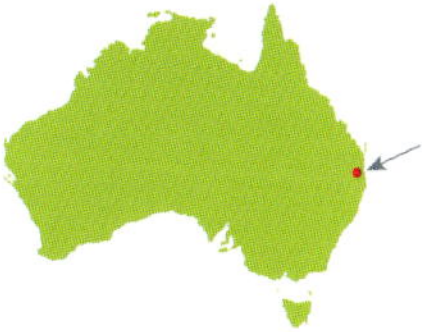

2–6mm long. Coppery brown head and body, darker tail. Aggressive, with a stinger on the tail. Introduced. Brisbane. Open areas such as lawns, along roads, paddocks. Inform your local council of the location of the ants so that they can eradicate them.

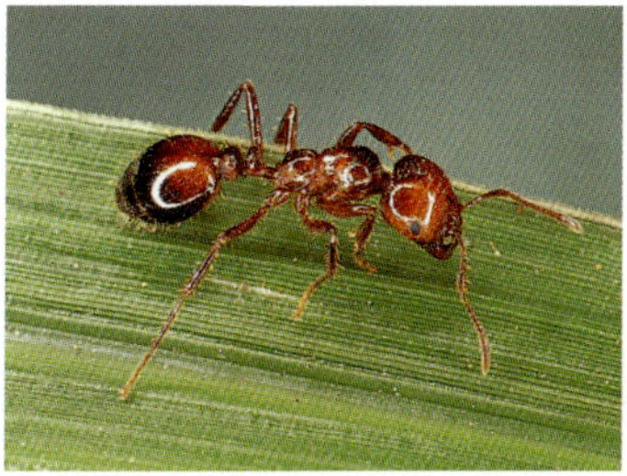

STEVE WILSON

Fire Ant worker

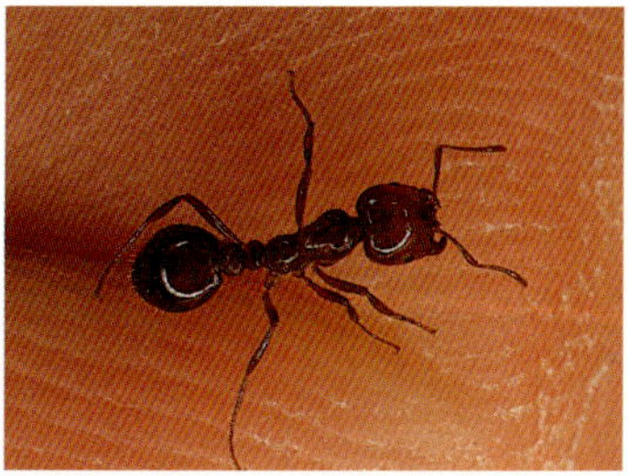

STEVE WILSON

Fire Ant soldier

Symptoms

A blister forms at the site of each fiery sting within a few hours. These become itchy as they heal. To avoid possible infection they should not be broken. If the victim is allergic to insect stings seek immediate medical attention.

First Aid

- Move victim away from ants and remove ants from their body.
- Apply ice pack/cold compress.
- Wash blisters with soap and water.
- If symptoms persist, seek medical aid.

MEAT ANT ★★

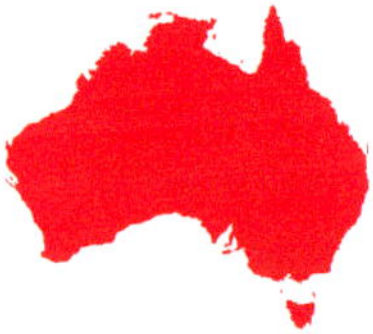

8–10mm long. Dark red with black abdomen. Large numbers around nest. These ants bite. Nests can be large, slightly raised mounds covered with small pebbles, or open, flat areas. Open bushland.

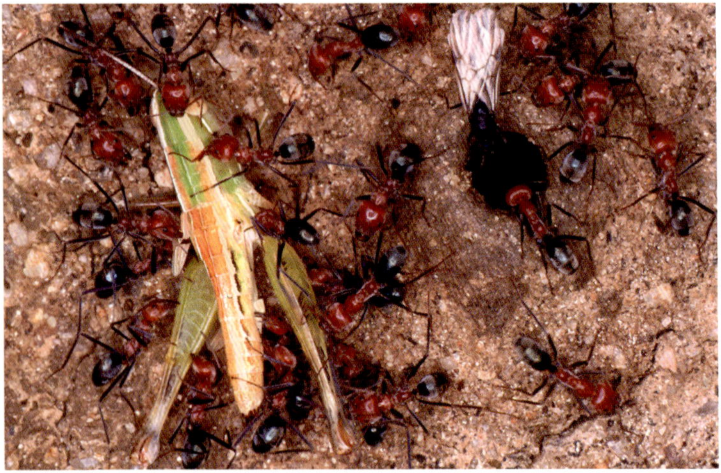

PAUL ZBOROWSKI

Symptoms

Sharp, painful sting.

First Aid

- Move the victim away from the ants and remove ants from their body.
- Apply ice pack/cold compress or calamine lotion.
- If symptoms persist, seek medical aid.

GREEN TREE ANT ★★

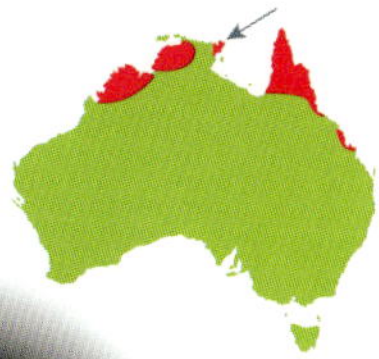

7–9mm long. Coppery head and body with green tail. These ants bind leaves together to build their nests in trees or tall shrubs. Bites usually occur when nests are disturbed and the ants drop onto the victim. Bushland.

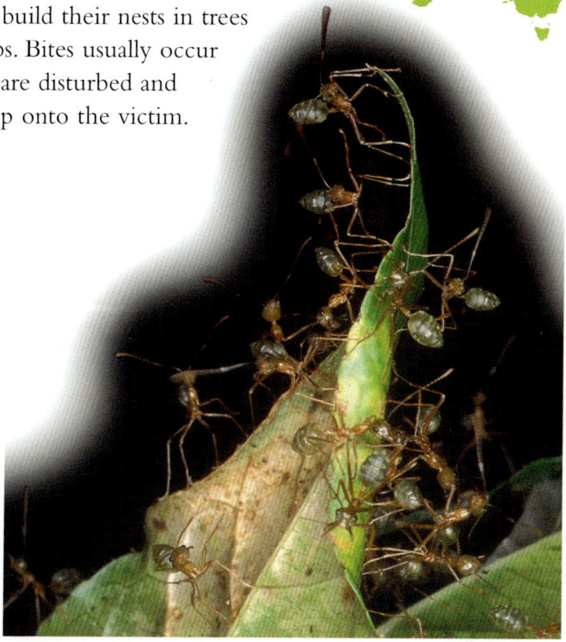

PAUL ZBOROWSKI

Symptoms

Sharp, painful sting.

First Aid

- Move victim away from ants and remove ants from their body.
- Apply ice pack/cold compress or calamine lotion.
- If symptoms persist, seek medical aid.

B BATS ★★★

(Flying Foxes, Fruit Bats, Microbats)

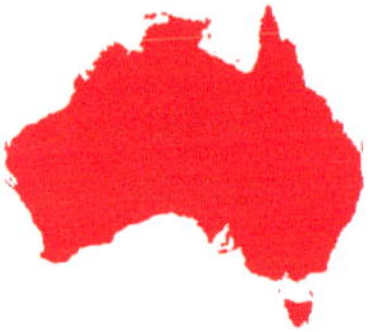

Tiny insect-eating microbats (from 31mm body length) to large Flying Foxes (up to 290mm body length). Fur-covered body with wings of thin skin. Microbats roost in hollows in trees, caves, crevices and buildings. Fruit bats roost in trees, sometimes in very large colonies.

Several species carry a virus (Australian bat lyssavirus) closely related to rabies that can be transmitted to people, and can be deadly. The virus is usually transmitted through bites and scratches. Avoid handling bats. If you must handle one, wear thick gloves. A vaccination is available for people who care for injured bats. Fruit bats are less widely distributed than others.

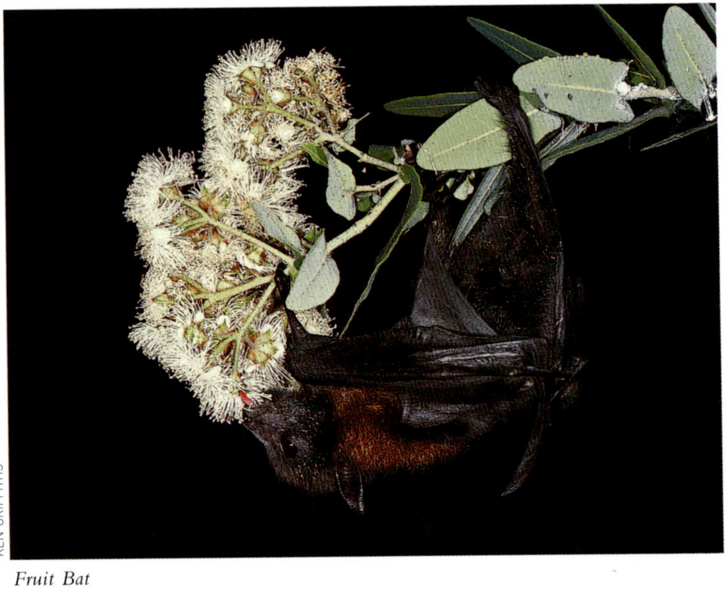

KEN GRIFFITHS

Fruit Bat

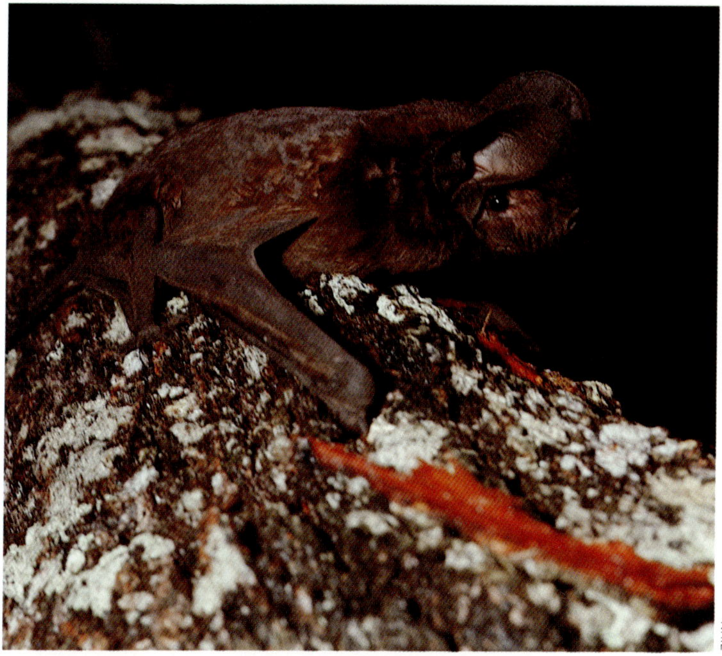
NHIL

Microbat

Symptoms

No immediate symptoms at time of bite, other than bite itself. However, symptoms ranging from fever, muscle pain, itching at site of healed bite, sore throat, choking and muscle spasms can appear at any time after bite.

First Aid

- Wash wound with soap and water for at least five minutes.
- Apply iodine after washing.
- Seek medical advice immediately.

B BEES ★★

MOST AUSTRALIAN native bees do not sting, but those that do can sting several times as there is no barb on their sting. Some are solitary and others have hives.

The introduced Honeybee, on the other hand, does have a barb at the end of its abdomen. The sting is caused by the bee embedding the barb into the skin. Once the bee has delivered its barb it cannot sting again and will die.

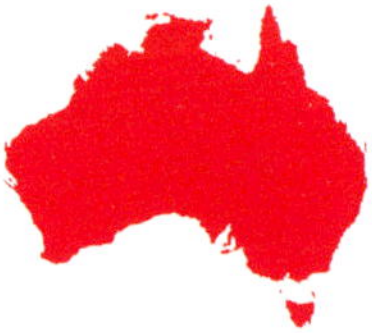

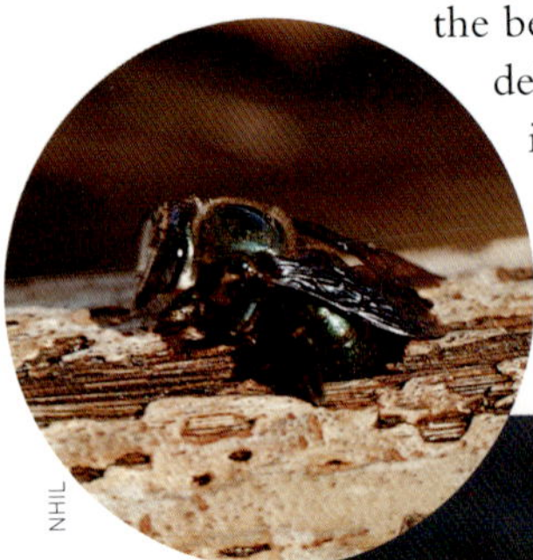

NHIL

Native bee

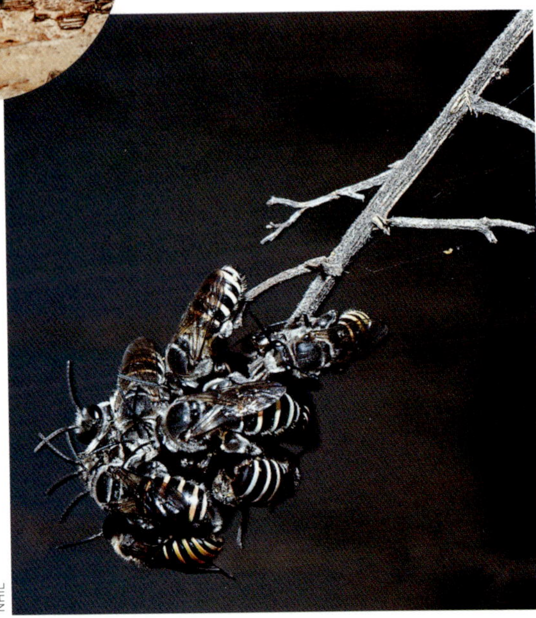

NHIL

Native bees clustering

HONEYBEE

(European Honeybee)

1–1.5cm long. Dark head, furry front of body, striped yellow and brown. Everywhere.

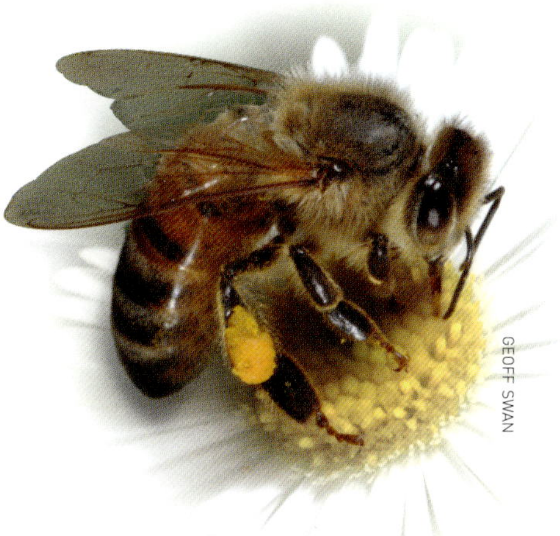

Symptoms

Painful sting. Swelling at site will usually subside after several hours. If there is an allergic reaction, swelling will continue to increase.

First Aid

- To remove barb, scrape barb sideways with a knife blade or fingernail. Do not grasp and try to pull out, as this will only squeeze more venom into the wound.
- Wash sting site, apply icepack/cold compress.
- Seek immediate medical assistance if allergic reaction occurs.

B BEETLES ★

SOME LARGER beetles (like those shown below) can give a painful nip with their jaws, but they are not dangerous. Others can give off a nasty smell or spray out a white vapour when disturbed. The beetle shown opposite can cause blisters.

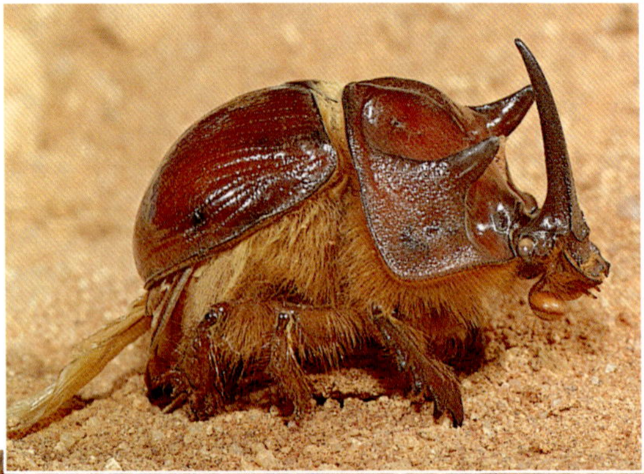

KEN GRIFFITHS

Rhinoceros beetle

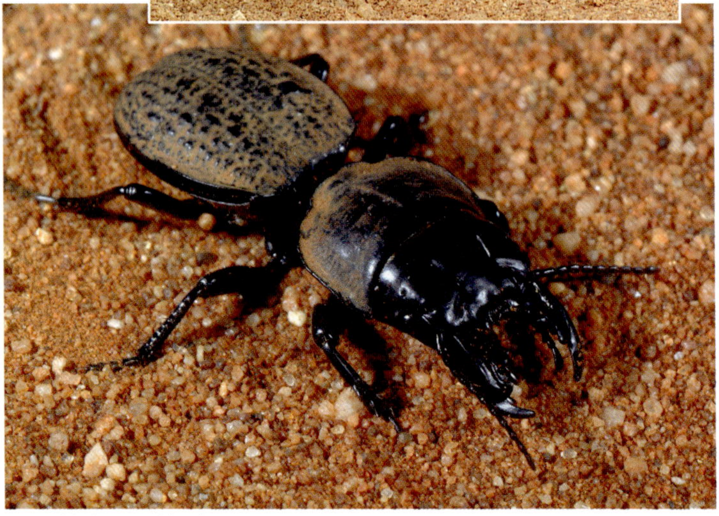

GEOFF SWAN

Large black ground beetle

WHIPLASH ROVE BEETLE

(Blister Beetle, Finch Hatton Bug)

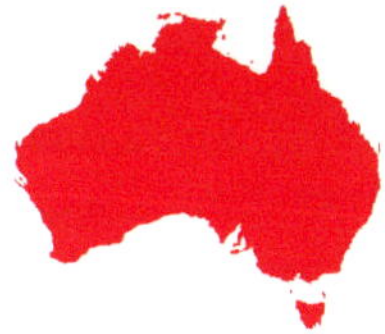

5–10mm long. Slender body, banded in blue–black and orange. Widespread. Live concealed on the ground, fly by night.

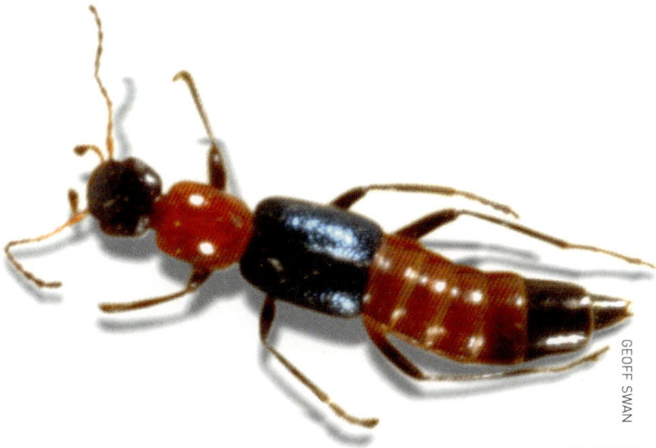

GEOFF SWAN

Symptoms

These beetles are attracted to houselights at night. They may drop onto the skin or into clothing, and when crushed release a contact poison. Because there are no immediate symptoms the delayed reaction is often not associated with the beetles. After 12 hours or more a red rash appears, then small blisters which become very painful and watery. These can get itchy when they start to heal.

First Aid

- Apply local anaesthetic cream to reduce pain and itchiness.
- When blisters break, apply antiseptic cream and a bandaid to prevent infection.

B BLUE-RINGED OCTOPUS ★★★★

(Blue-banded Octopus, Spotted Octopus)

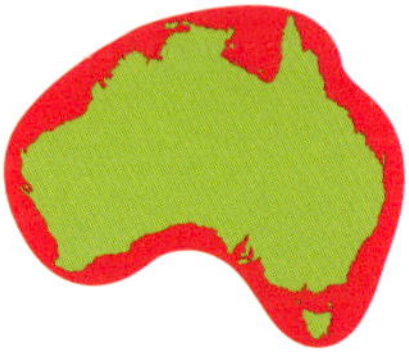

2–20cm across outspread tentacles. Normally yellow–brown with darker markings. Merges into background colouration. When disturbed or excited the markings become a vivid, iridescent blue. Coastal waters. Live in shells, in rock pools, under rock ledges or wherever they find a good hiding place.

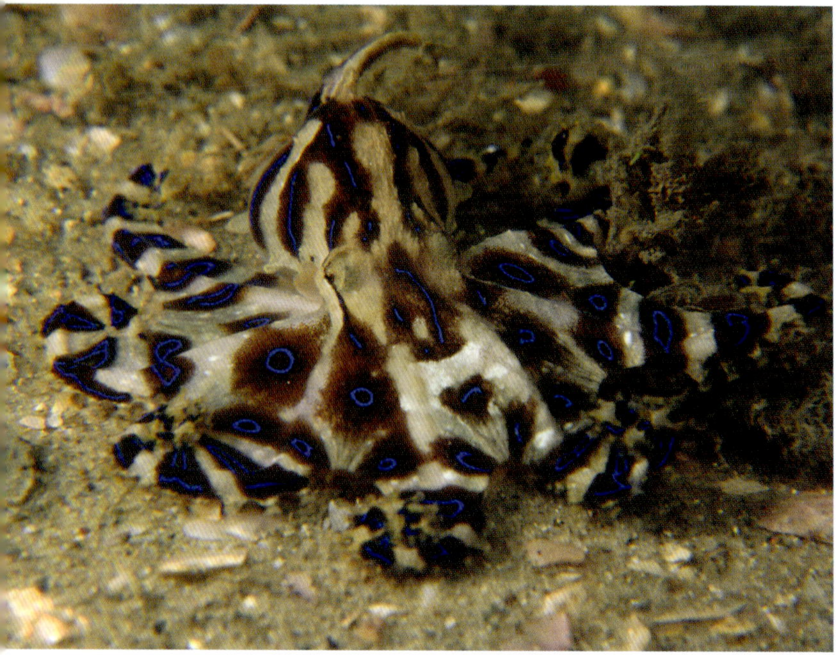

NEIL VINCENT

BLUE-RINGED OCTOPUS

B

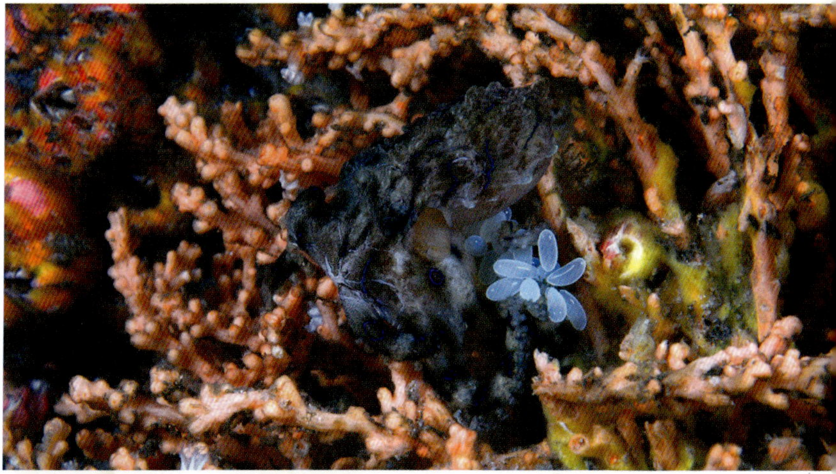

BECCA SAUNDERS

Blue-ringed Octopuses are well camouflaged when inactive—the blue rings aren't visible.

Symptoms

An octopus caught and handled will bite with its small parrot-like beak, which is located underneath the body. You may not notice the actual bite as it is almost painless. However, symptoms are apparent within minutes: tingling and numbness around mouth; difficulty swallowing, speaking and breathing; and blurred vision. These can progress to partial or complete muscular paralysis, no breathing and death.

First Aid

- If paralysis has not occurred, wash wound, apply a pressure bandage (see page 15), keep victim still and send for medical assistance.
- If paralysis has occurred, commence EAR immediately (see page 11) and if necessary, CPR (see page 12). Send for medical assistance.

B BRISTLE WORMS ★★

(Beachworms, Giant Beachworms, Biting Reef Worms, Sea Mice, Fireworms, Kingworms, Greenheads, Bronzeheads, Bullworms, Hairy Marys)

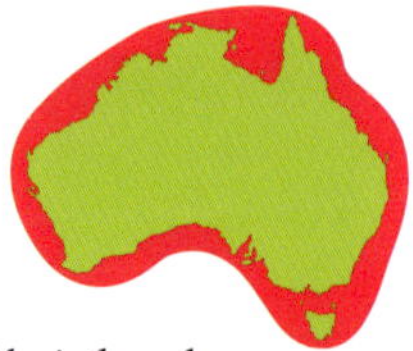

5–150cm long. Typically with rows or tufts of bristles along body. Many are colourful. Bristle worms belong to a group of animals called segmented worms that includes the earthworm. Coastal waters. Burrow into sand, hide under rocks or in coral.

Beachworms can bite but don't sting.

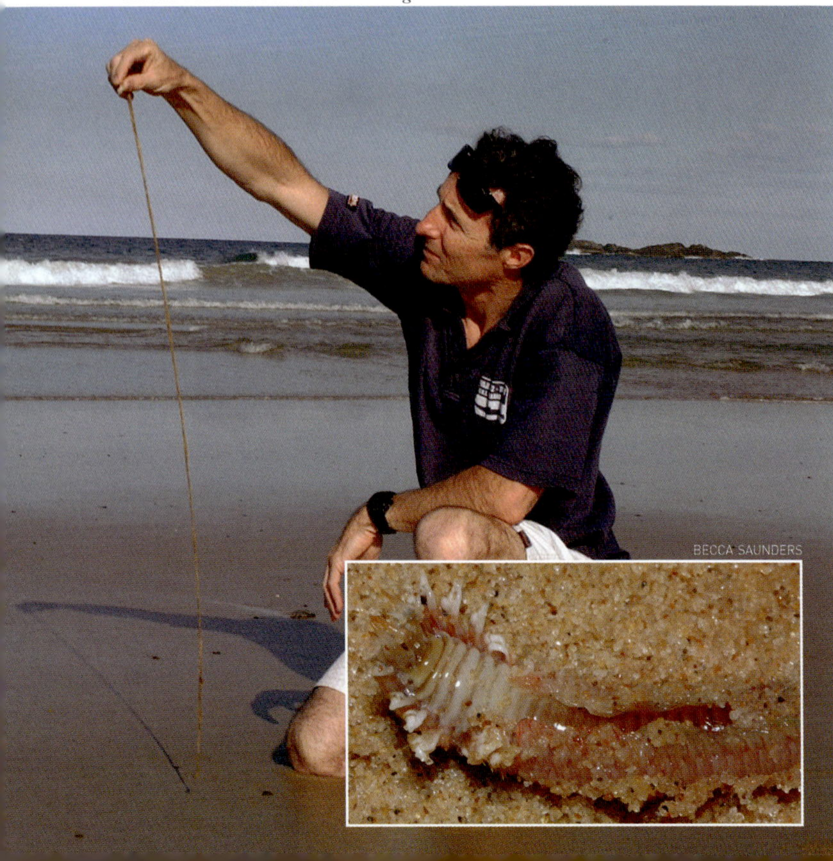

BECCA SAUNDERS

BECCA SAUNDERS

BRISTLE WORMS

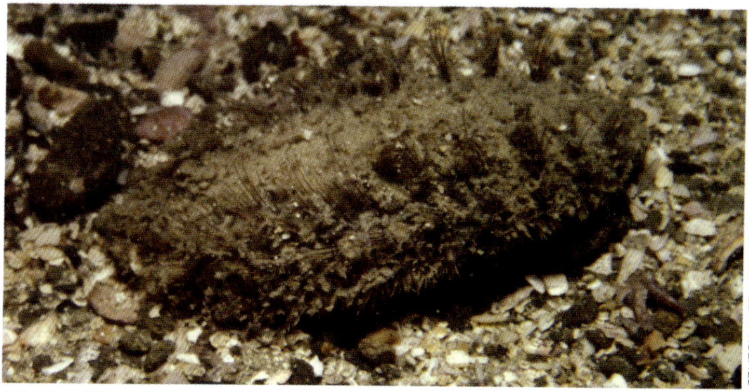

The Sea Mouse has stinging bristles.

Symptoms

Some bristle worms can bite; they can also puncture skin with their bristles. Bites quickly become hot, swollen and inflamed. Contact with the bristles may cause them to penetrate the skin and break off, resulting in itching or burning, pain and swelling, with blisters developing. The effect of a bite can last up to two days, the bristles up to 10 days.

First Aid

Bites

- Wash with salt water or antiseptic.

Bristles

- Remove by rubbing with sand or placing sticking plaster or adhesive tape over the area and pulling off.
- Apply cooling calamine lotion or methylated spirits and/or antibiotic ointment.
- Seek medical aid if symptoms (of bites or bristles) persist.

BUGS ★

BUGS DIFFER from beetles in having a specialised mouth. This consists of a series of sharp tubes for piercing and sucking. While bugs are not dangerous, several can cause painful or irritating bites.

ASSASSIN BUG

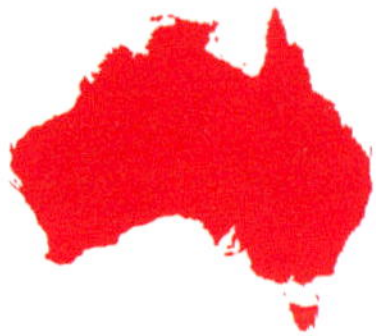

7–30mm long. Recognisable by the large curved 'beak' which they can use to inflict a painful bite. Many are brightly coloured, making them attractive to children. Bushland, gardens.

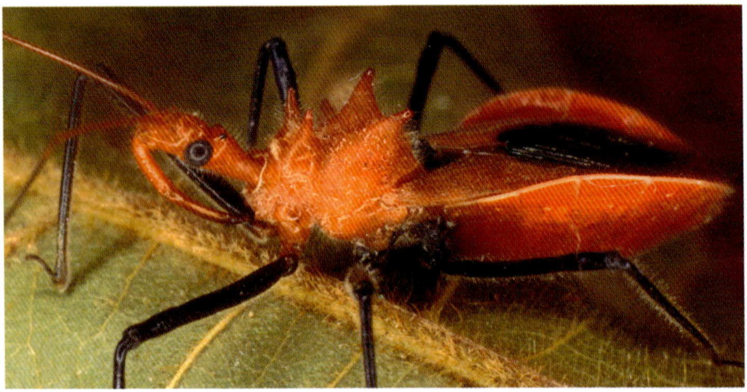

PAUL ZBOROWSKI

Symptoms
Sharp local pain at time of bite. May last for a few minutes.

First Aid
- Remove bug and wash bite.

FISH-KILLER BUG

(Toe Biter, Water Scorpion, Great Water Bug)

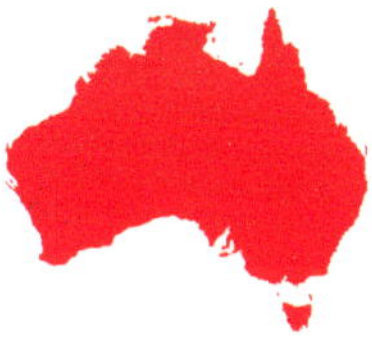

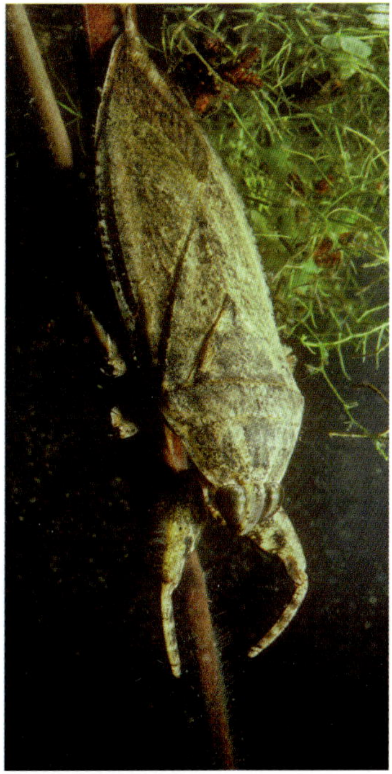

PAUL ZBOROWSKI

4–7cm long. Flattened shield shape, with well-developed wings and flattened, fringed legs for swimming. Front legs are designed to grasp prey. A long breathing siphon extends from the rear. Ponds and other water bodies. Swimming pools.

Symptoms

The straight, long tail which gives this bug its name is not a sting. The bite is inflicted by the beak-like mouth. Known to sometimes bite swimmers or the toe of a person wading barefoot through muddy water. Sharp local pain for a few minutes.

First Aid

- Wash wound. Apply antiseptic cream if bite occurred in dirty water.

BED BUG

(Stink Bug, Backpacker Bug)

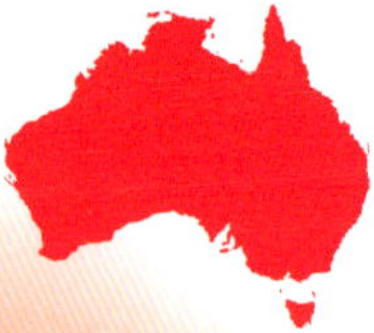

5–7mm long. Flattened, almost round, reddish brown and wingless. Houses. Introduced into Australia with European settlement.

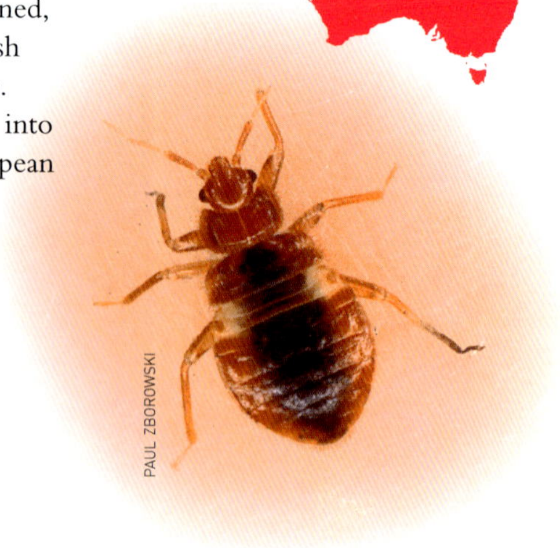

PAUL ZBOROWSKI

Symptoms

Irritating bites during the night. Local swelling and itching. Scratching the bites could lead to infection.

With today's improved standards of hygiene Bed Bugs are seldom reported. They hide during the day in cracks and crevices, emerging at night to suck blood from the victim. More recently they have picked up the name of Backpacker Bugs because they hitch a ride into Australia in the folds and pockets of backpacking luggage.

First Aid

- Apply calamine lotion to reduce itchiness.
- Avoid scratching itchy area.
- If infection occurs, seek medical aid.

CITRUS BUG

(Stink Bug, Bronze Orange Bug)

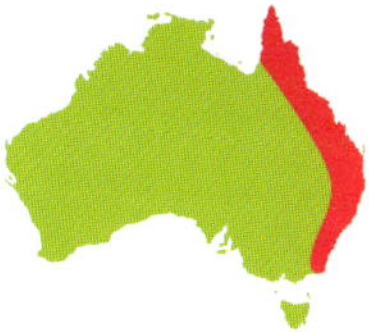

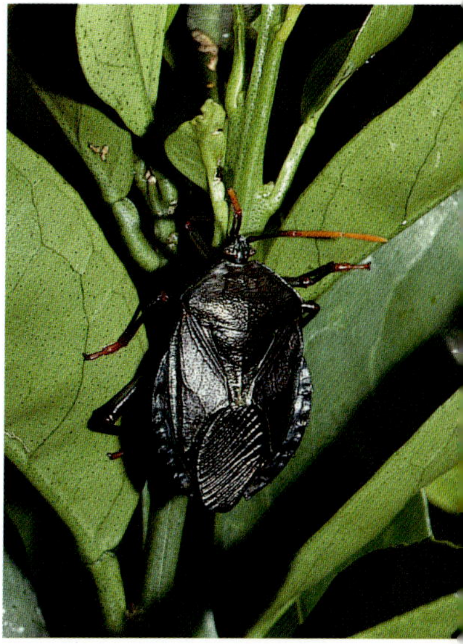

DENISE GREIG

25mm long. Stoutly built. Bronze, becoming black with age. Legs and part of antennae are red. Emits a foul odour and corrosive secretions. Can squirt liquid up to 60cm. A pest of citrus trees, eating new foliage. Can gather in big clusters on a tree.

Symptoms

Squirted liquid can cause a stinging, burning sensation on skin as well as staining it.

First Aid

On skin

- Wash with soap and water and apply a local anaesthetic ointment if necessary.

In eyes

- Wash eyes with copious amounts of water. Seek medical aid if discomfort continues.

C CANE TOAD ★★

(Giant Toad)

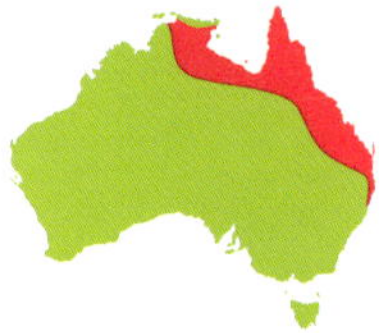

10–25cm long. Tan with dark brown blotches. Very warty, with a pair of prominent glands behind neck. Toxic white secretion from glands on neck can be sprayed to a distance of 2m. A bony ridge above each eye extends to the snout, where they meet. Sometimes large native frogs (see opposite) are mistaken for Cane Toads and killed. Bushland, urban.

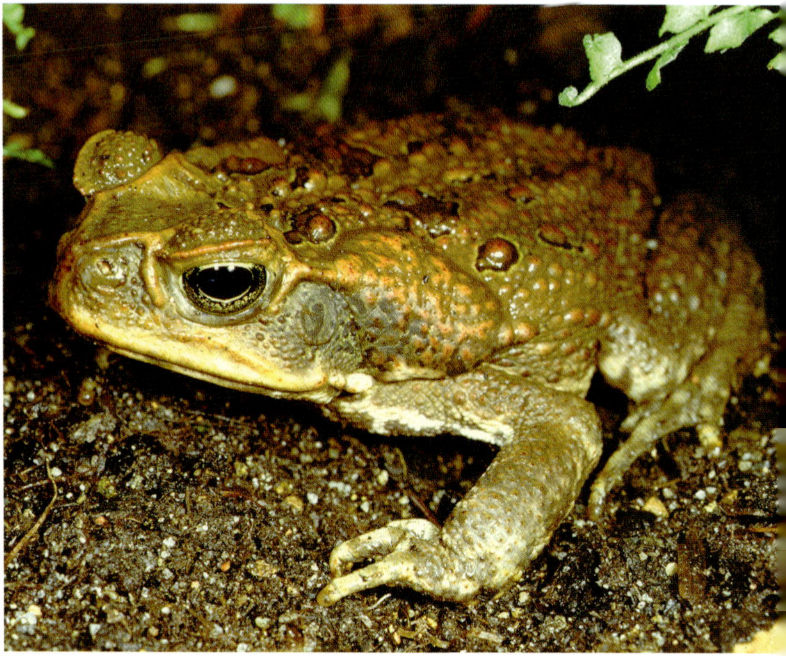

GEOFF SWAN

The introduced Cane Toad is the only true toad in Australia. It was imported in the mistaken belief that it would control Sugar Cane Beetles. The toad itself is now a pest, with disastrous consequences for native wildlife.

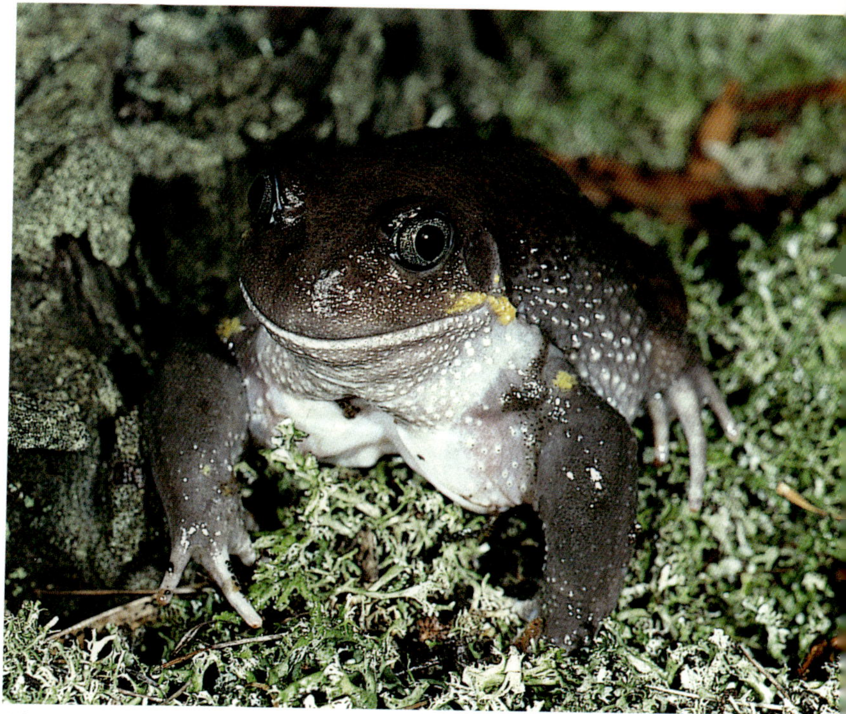

KEN GRIFFITHS

The Giant Burrowing Frog is sometimes mistaken for a Cane Toad and killed.

Symptoms

Severe pain if the white secretion from the glands on the back gets into the eyes, mouth or open wounds.

First Aid

- If a toad has been handled, wash hands thoroughly.
- If secretion has got into eyes, wash with lots of running water.

C CATERPILLARS ★★

MOST CATERPILLARS are completely harmless but a few can sting. Avoid those that have hairs or bristles on the back.

CUP MOTH CATERPILLAR

(Slug Caterpillars, Chinese Junks)

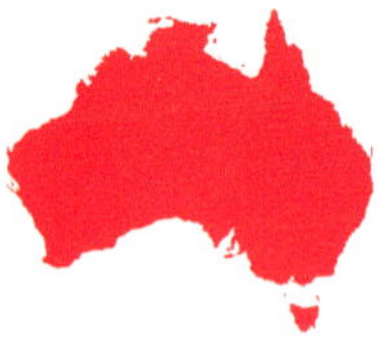

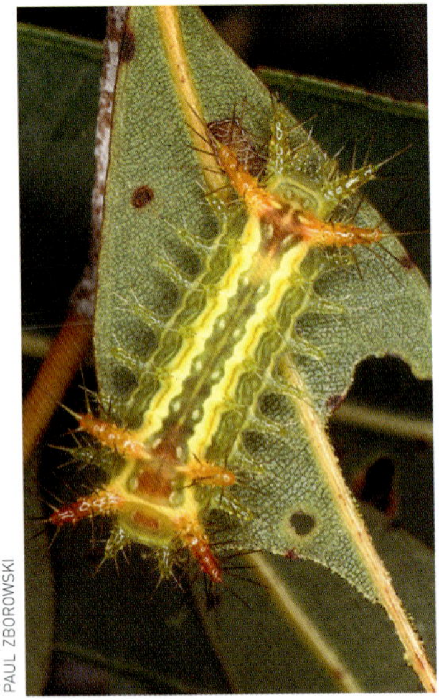

PAUL ZBOROWSKI

2–3cm long. Bright green, yellow and red with clusters of bristles on the back. Widespread. Bushland, urban.

Symptoms

If the bristles are touched they embed into the skin and a poison passes up the bristle and into the skin, causing stinging and itching. A raised red mark or rash may develop.

First Aid

- To remove bristles, cover with a bandaid or adhesive tape then pull the tape off. Repeat as necessary.
- Apply calamine lotion to ease the stinging.
- Seek medical attention if an allergic reaction occurs.

PROCESSIONARY CATERPILLAR

(Bagworm)

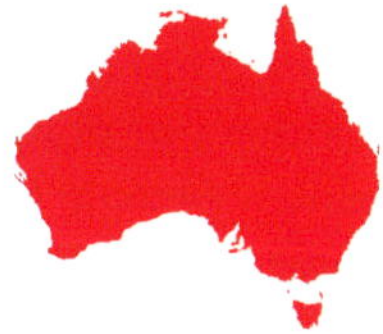

2–3cm long. Covered in hairs. Sometimes seen on the ground moving along in a procession. Widespread. Bushland, urban.

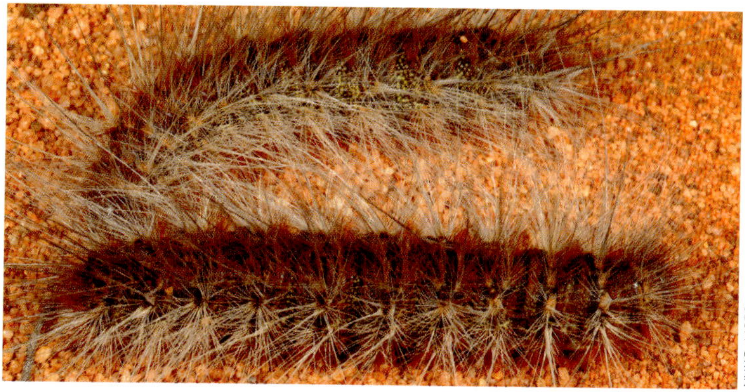

GEOFF SWAN

Symptoms

Barbed hairs break off on contact and are embedded into the skin, causing stinging and itching. A raised red mark or rash may develop. In some species the hairs become detached from the caterpillar and blow about in the wind or fall to the ground, and will sting on contact.

First Aid

- To remove bristles, cover with a bandaid or adhesive tape then pull the tape off. Repeat as necessary.
- Apply calamine lotion to ease the stinging.
- Seek medical attention if an allergic reaction occurs.

C CENTIPEDES ★★

3–15cm long. Various colours, such as tan, brown, blue, yellow, orange or green. Flattened body divided into many segments, each with a pair of legs sticking out from the side. Tail appendage is harmless; obvious fangs are located on head. Centipedes are sometimes confused with millipedes. However, millipedes have a cylindrical body, no obvious fangs and small legs underneath the body. Shelter under rocks, logs or debris, usually in moist spots, during the day and come out at night. Bushland, urban.

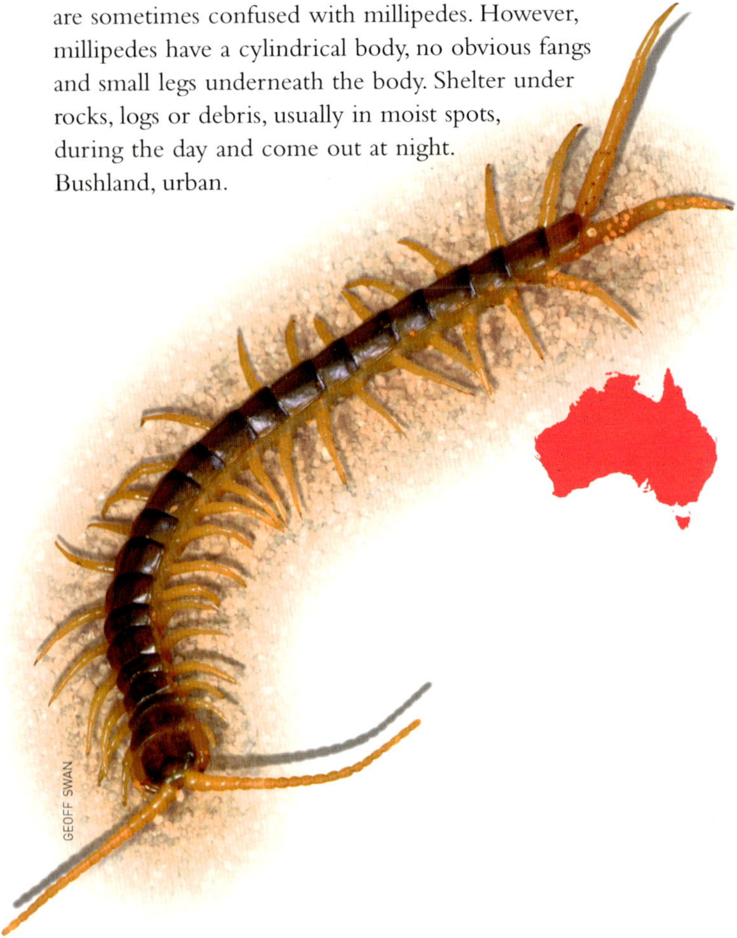

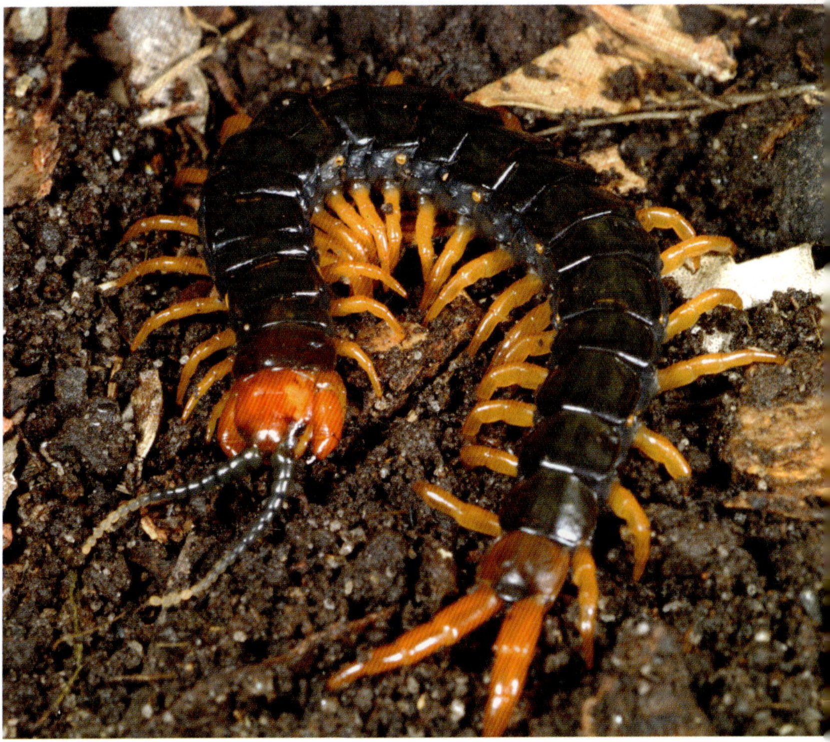

GEOFF SWAN

Symptoms

Immediate, sometimes intense, burning sensation. Swelling and throbbing, which may last for a day or more.

First Aid

- Apply ice pack/cold compress.
- If symptoms persist, or the bite is on the face, seek medical aid.

C CRABS ★

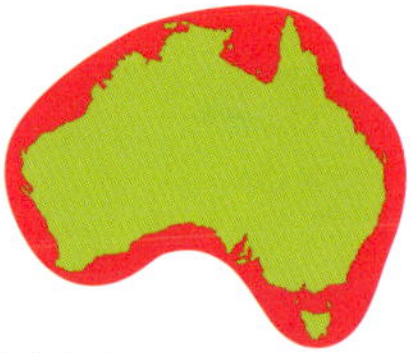

2–400mm wide. All shapes, sizes and colours. All are covered in a hard shell, have a pair of claws, four pairs of walking legs (they walk sideways) and eyes on stalks. Some crabs are poisonous to eat but describing these is beyond the scope of this book. Almost all live in or near sea water but two live in freshwater streams. Around the coastline on sandy beaches, in rock pools and in the water.

NHIL

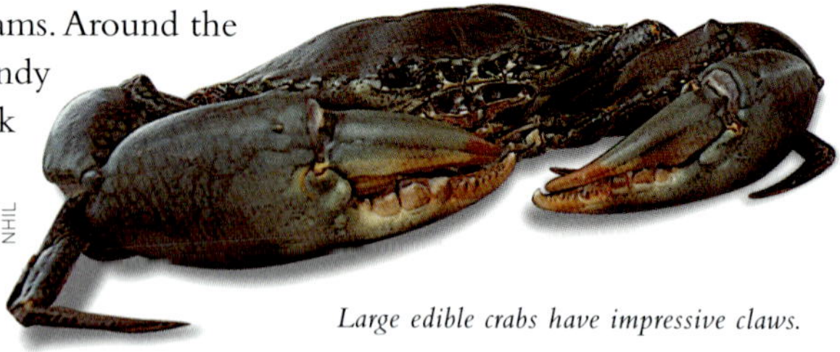

Large edible crabs have impressive claws.

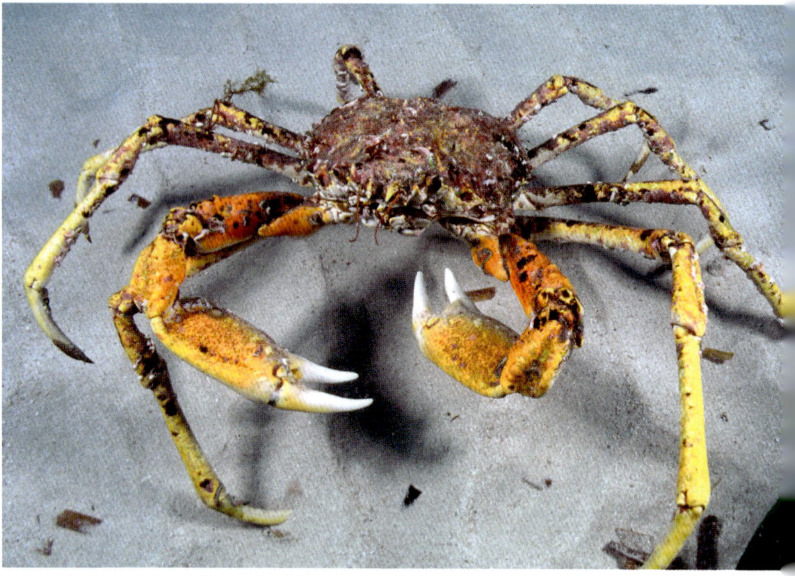

BECCA SAUNDERS

Giant Spider Crab

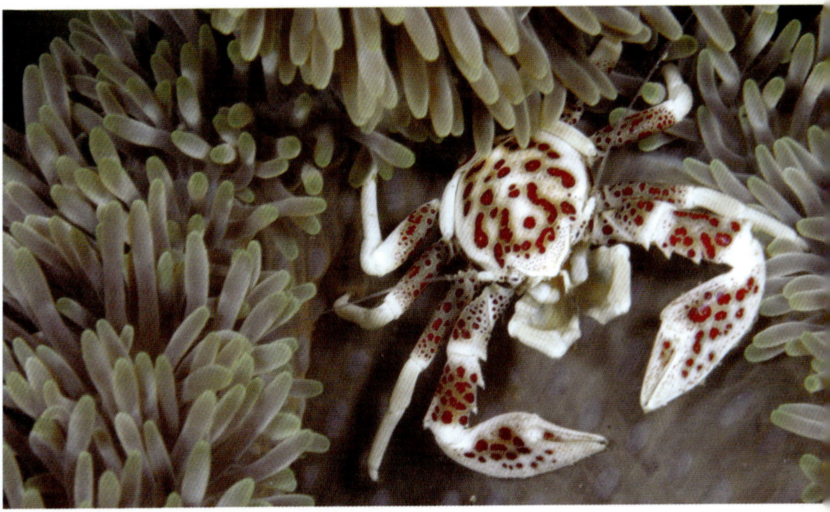

SANDY JACKA

Anemone Crab

Symptoms

Most crabs will give no more than a painful nip if molested. Large crabs can clamp a claw onto a finger, hand or foot, causing a painful, crushing injury. The claw can break off the crab and still remain firmly attached to the victim.

First Aid

- Remove crab. If claw has become detached from crab, prize apart or smash the joint of the claw, taking care not to further injure victim.
- Apply ice pack/cold compress to reduce pain.
- Disinfect if skin broken as injuries from sea creatures tend to get infected.
- Seek medical aid if there is a possibility of broken or crushed bones.

C CROCODILES

TWO SPECIES of crocodile are found in Australia: the Saltwater or Estuarine Crocodile and the Freshwater or Johnstone's Crocodile. Only the Estuarine Crocodile is regarded as dangerous, but the Freshwater Crocodile can and will bite if molested, and is capable of inflicting a nasty wound. Crocodiles feed during the day but are most active at night. Estuarine Crocodiles will lie in wait underwater close to shore and lunge out to seize prey. People are no exception.

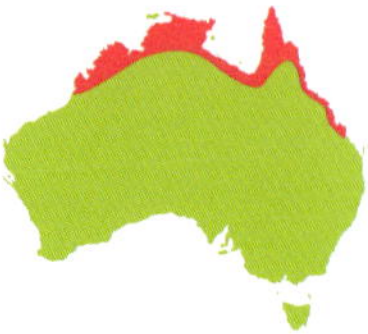

ESTUARINE CROCODILE ★★★★

(Saltwater Crocodile)

3–7m long. Broad, blunt snout. Coastal rivers, swamps and estuaries, extending inland up the major rivers. Individuals are occasionally seen swimming in the ocean or moving along the coast.

Right: Typical crocodile habitat, especially for 'Salties'.

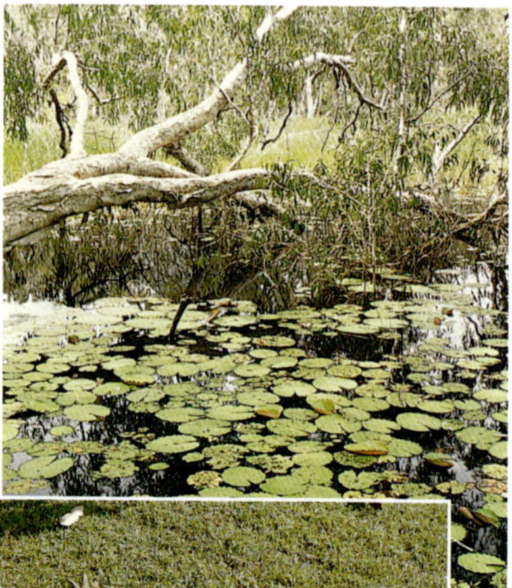

ROB VALENTIC

Below: Saltie in a wildlife park.

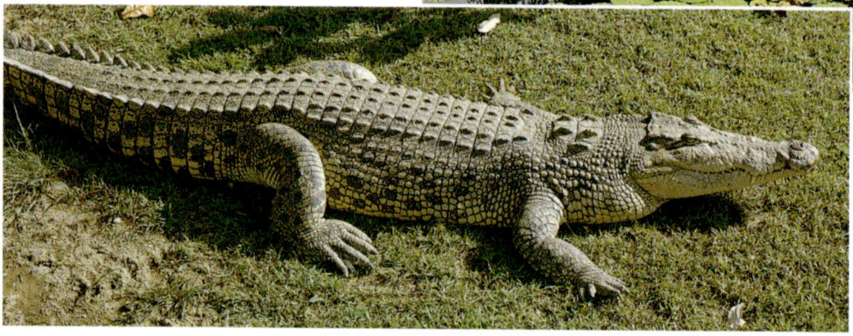

NHIL

FRESHWATER CROCODILE ★★★

(Johnstone's Crocodile)

2–3m long. Long, slim snout.
Freshwater rivers and billabongs.

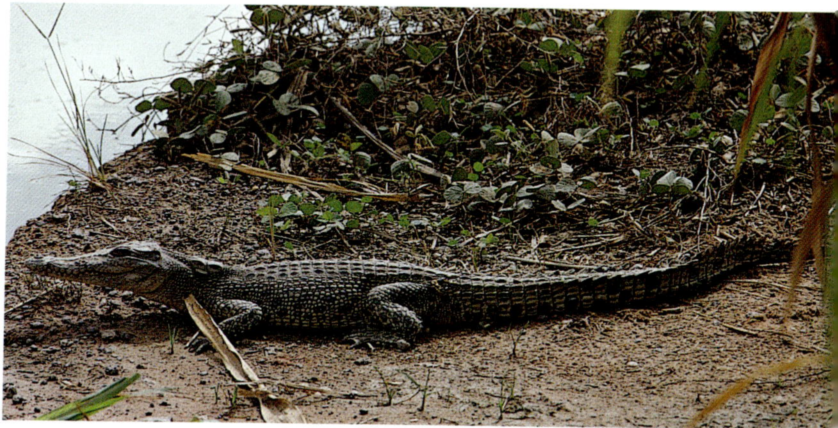

The snout of a 'Freshie' is long and thin compared with that of a Saltie.

Symptoms

A crocodile bite will most probably result in severe injuries and blood loss, and in the case of the Estuarine Crocodile, death. The victim may go into shock.

First Aid

- It's vital that you stop the bleeding as quickly as possible (see page 14).
- Treat victim for shock (see page 16).
- Seek medical attention urgently.

C CROWN-OF-THORNS STARFISH ★★★

(Sea Star, Venomous Starfish)

Up to 60cm in diameter. Only known venomous starfish. Has 13–16 arms compared with the usual five arms on most starfish. The top is covered in sharp spines up to 6cm long. Feeds on live corals and is responsible for killing areas of the Great Barrier Feef. Found on coral reefs.

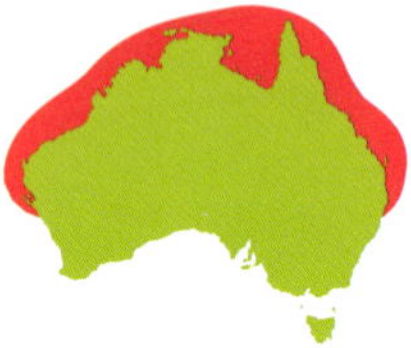

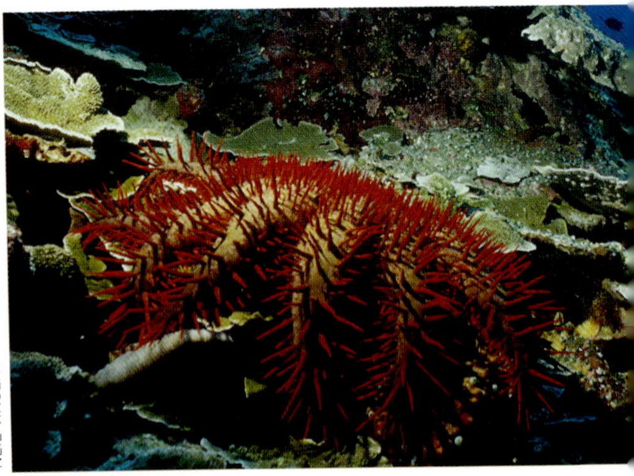

NEIL VINCENT

Symptoms

Injuries usually occur when divers touch or brush against the spines, which can become embedded in the skin, causing immediate, severe pain. There may be vomiting, as well as swelling and numbness that can last for several days.

First Aid

- Pull out loose spines carefully with fingers, tweezers or pliers as they can break off easily. Do not wiggle them around, just pull straight out. Leave any embedded spines for a doctor to remove.
- Immerse affected area in hot water to relieve pain.
- Seek medical aid immediately to make sure no spines remain embedded in the skin as these could cause infection.

DOGS COME in all sizes and with many temperaments. Dog owners have a responsibility to make sure their dogs are well trained keep them under control. Do not move towards or touch any dog that you don't know, particularly if the dog is not on a lead. Teach children how to behave towards dogs. Stay away from feral dogs and dingos and do not offer them food.

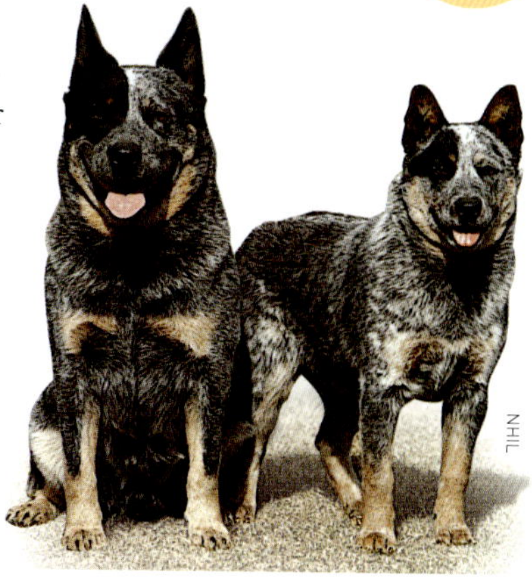
NHIL

Symptoms

A dog bite may involve puncture wounds and gashes which can easily become infected as dogs tend to carry a lot of germs in their mouths. A tetanus shot may be necessary.

First Aid

Minor bites

- Carefully wash wound with water and antiseptic or soap.
- Apply an ice pack/cold compress to reduce swelling.
- Apply antiseptic and cover with a dressing.
- Check the wound each day for any redness or tenderness that could indicate an infection. If this occurs see a doctor.
- Dog bites on the face, particularly in children, require medical attention to prevent infection and scarring.

Severe bites

- Your first priority is to stop the bleeding as quickly as possible (see page 14).
- Seek medical attention.

E EELS ★★★

(Moray eels, conger eels, freshwater eels)

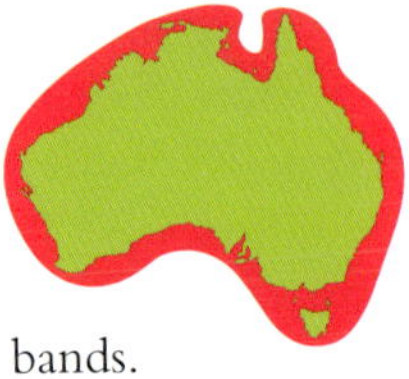

0.2–3m long. Snake-like but without the flattened tail of the sea snakes. Although most are drab coloured, many of the moray eels are brightly coloured, often with spots or bands.

There are many types of eels, and all should be treated with respect. Moray and conger eels are found in salt water, while freshwater eels, as the name suggests, spend most of their lives in fresh water. These three are the ones you're most likely to encounter around the coast in rivers, streams and dams, often in crevices or among rocks.

Eels usually attack because of intrusion into their territory or because they are being molested or have been injured. But with the increase in the number of people going diving, and the popularity of hand-feeding moray eels, there can be a problem if these eels are approached and food not supplied.

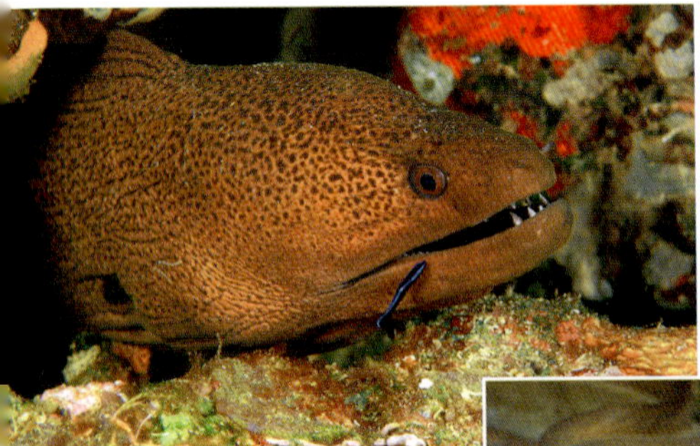

BECCA SAUNDERS

Moray eel

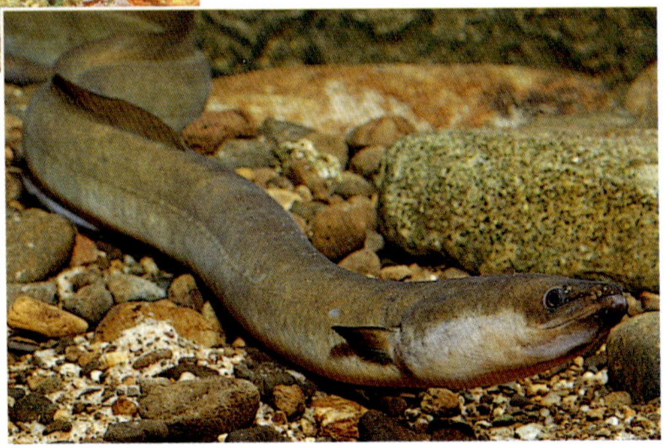

GUNTHER SCHMIDA/LT

Freshwater eel

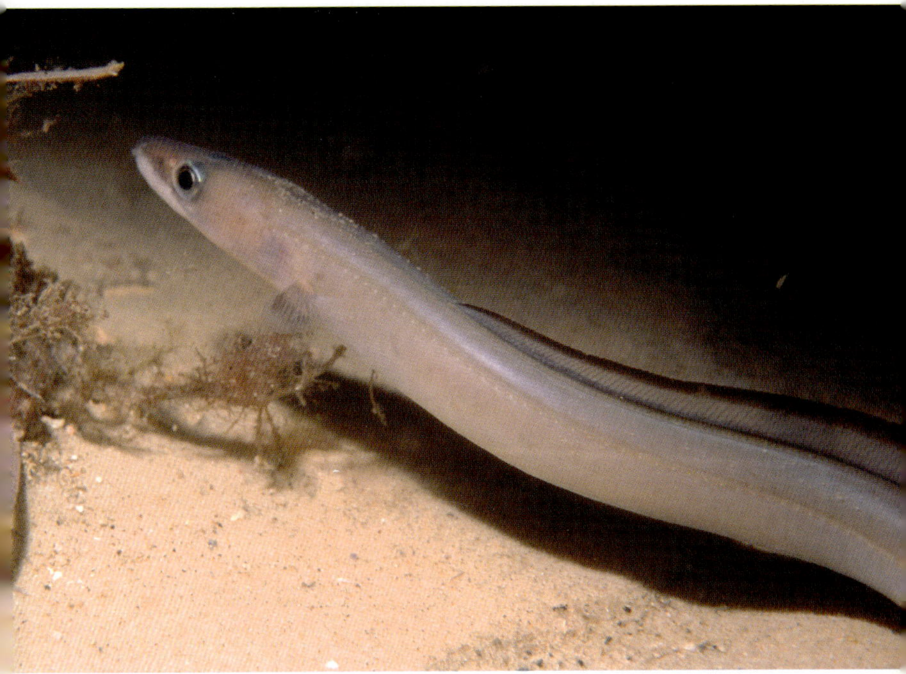

Short-finned conger eel ERIK SCHLOGL

Symptoms

Ragged, torn bite with copious bleeding. Freshwater eel bites are not usually serious.

First Aid

- Remove victim from water and reassure.
- Lay victim down and keep them comfortable and warm.
- Your priority is to stop the bleeding (see page 14).
- Seek medical attention.

E ELECTRIC RAYS ★★★

(Numbfish, Coffin Ray, Torpedo Ray, Numb Ray)

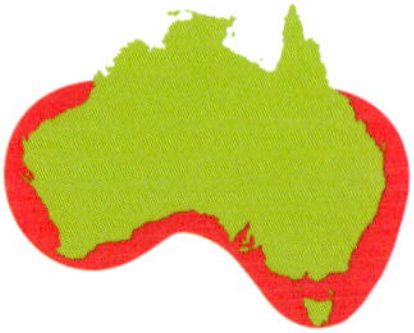

20–60cm long. Flattened oblong body with eyes on top of head. Tail is short and, unlike stingrays, has no spine. Uses an electric shock to subdue prey or to protect itself. Can deliver a series of shocks, lessening in intensity, on being touched or trodden on, even if the ray is out of water. There are reports of the electric shock travelling up wet fishing line. They are slow swimmers, usually found submerged in mud or sand in coastal waters south of the Tropic of Capricorn.

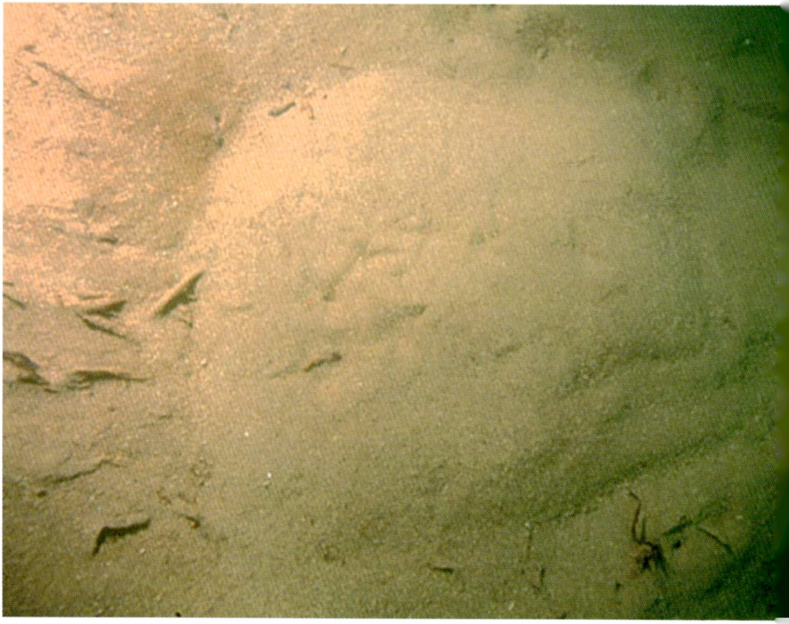

ERIK SCHLOGL

Numbfish buried in sand

ELECTRIC RAYS

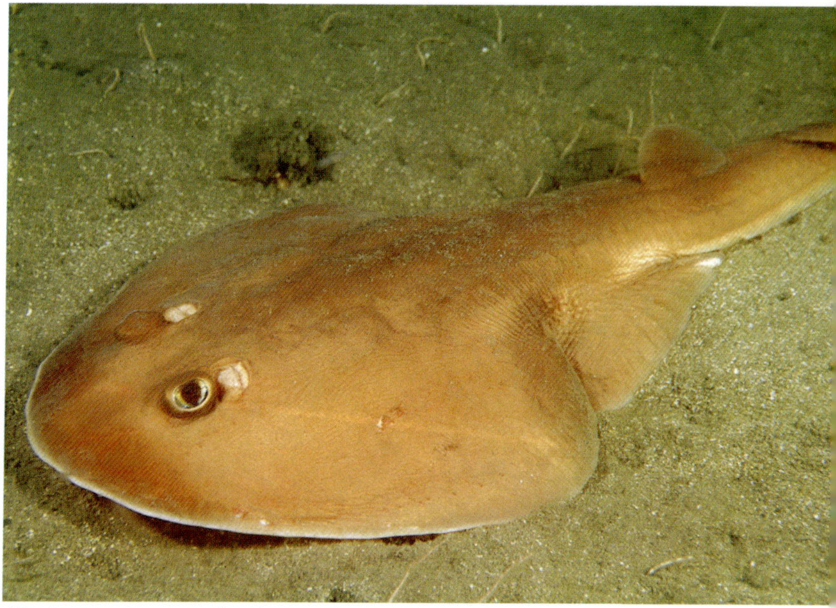

MARINETHEMES.COM/KELVIN AITKEN

Electric ray resting on sea floor

Symptoms

Mild electric shock can cause tingling; stronger shock may be capable of knocking down and temporarily disabling a person, with the danger of drowning.

First Aid

- If the victim is in the water they may need to be rescued and resuscitated using EAR or CPR (see pages 11–12).
- Treatment not usually required for the electric shock.

F FIRE CORAL ★

(Stinging Coral, Itching Coral)

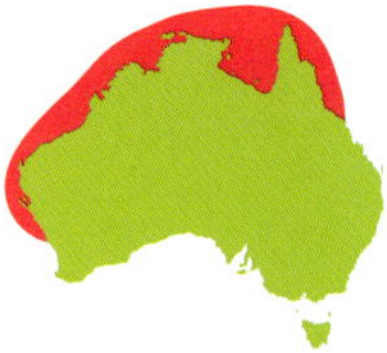

Fire Coral is similar to true coral but softer. Occurring in many different shapes and colours, it can be fern- or sponge-like and is usually brown or yellow–green in colour. Uses stinging cells to capture microscopic organisms in the sea.

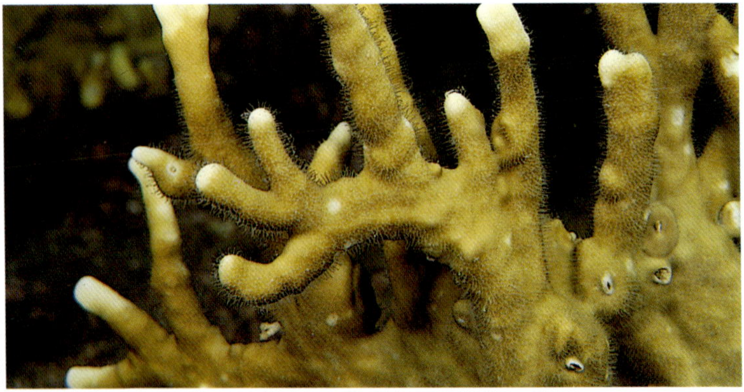

BECCA SAUNDERS

Symptoms

Brushing against corals may result in stinging cells penetrating the skin, causing itchiness and a painful burning sensation, and often red lesions, weals and swelling.

First Aid

- Remove victim from the water and reassure.
- Lay victim down and keep them comfortable and warm.
- Use a local anaesthetic ointment to reduce pain. If this is not available immerse the area in hot water or cover with a hot pack.
- Seek medical aid.

FIRE WEED ★

(Stinging Seaweed, Fire Fern)

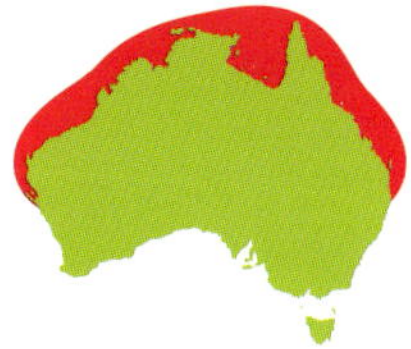

Up to 30cm long. Seaweed-like animals, some with branches like cypress trees and others quite feathery. Equipped with stinging cells that can penetrate the skin and cause extreme discomfort. Green, brown, white or purple, usually attached to rocks. Coral reefs in tropical waters.

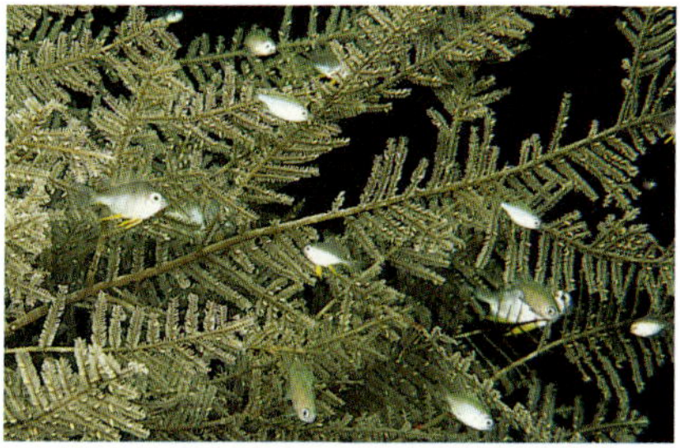

BECCA SAUNDERS

Juvenile fish hide among fire weed fronds.

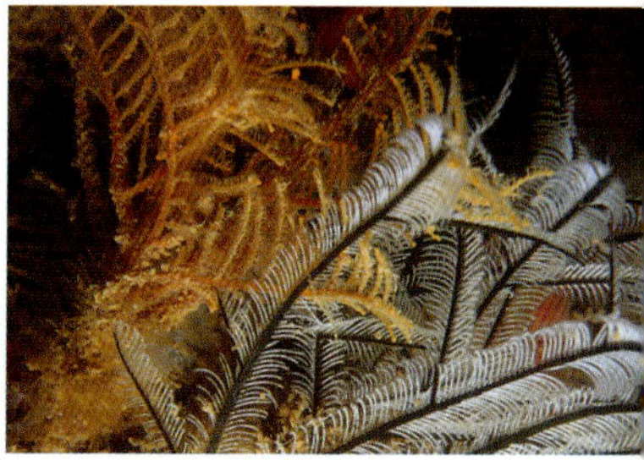

NEIL VINCENT

Fire Weed

Symptoms

Sometimes cause extreme pain when touched, but inexplicably at other times there is no effect. Mild stinging to severe pain, increasing over 10–15 minutes. The stung area becomes blotchy red with weals.

First Aid

- Remove victim from the water and reassure.
- Lay victim down and keep them comfortable and warm.
- Wash the affected area gently with water.
- Use a local anaesthetic ointment to reduce pain.

F FISH

MARINE ANIMALS are diverse and have developed a range of spines, stings, teeth and darts, many with poisons. Few of these animals are dangerous, but a surprising range of fish have spines which can penetrate the skin and inject venom. Spines may be around the fins, head or tail. In some species they are quite obvious, in others they are concealed until the animal is threatened. Some of the very dangerous fish, plus a few others, are included here, but it is not possible to include every fish that might sting. Apart from those shown in this book, others to be aware of include: Goblinfish, Port Jackson Shark (Doggie), South Australian Cobbler, and Gurnard Perch.

Venomous fish wounds display similar symptoms, but differ in the severity and duration of the pain. Current first-aid treatment is essentially the same for all species.

First Aid

- Remove victim from water, lay them down, immobilise and reassure them.
- Keep victim comfortable and warm.
- Wash wound and if possible remove any remaining spines with tweezers or fingers.
- Immerse limb in hot water (taking care not to scald victim) or apply heat in other ways (e.g. hot sand) to relieve pain.
- Treat for shock if necessary (see page 16).
- Seek immediate medical aid.
- If victim loses consciousness and stops breathing, commence EAR (see page 11) immediately and, if necessary, CPR (see page 12).

STONEFISH ★★★★

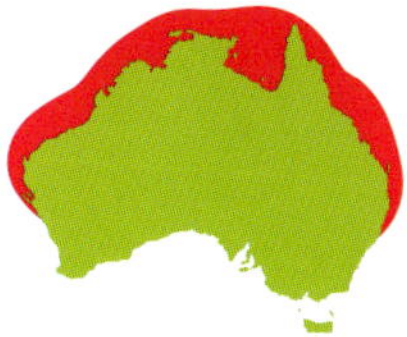

20–30cm long. Ugly, with warty lumps on the body, no scales, grotesque head, 13 dorsal fin spines. Burrows into mud and sand where it lies perfectly camouflaged. Coastline.

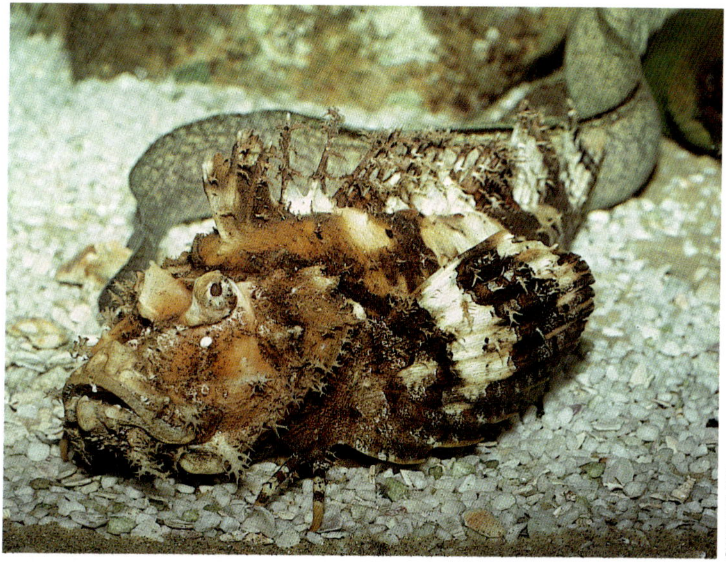

KEN GRIFFITHS

Symptoms (First Aid — see page 54)

The most venomous fish known—the sting can result in death. An antivenom is available. Puncture wound with immediate pain, increasing rapidly in intensity until it becomes excruciating. Victim may lose consciousness. Pain lessens after a few hours but may last for days. Wound becomes swollen, hot, numb at centre but very tender at edges. Tissue around wound becomes red or bluish.

DEVIL FISH ★★★

(Bearded Ghoul, Demon Stinger)

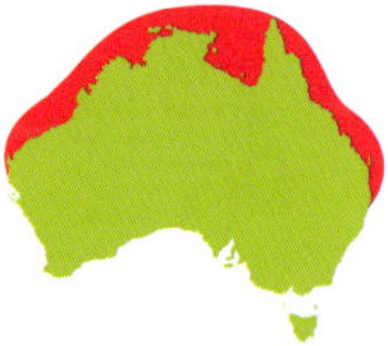

Up to 30cm long. Like the Stonefish, this is a grotesque-looking animal with 17 strong spines along the back. Normally found in deep water but sometimes comes into estuaries and rivers. Sub-tropical and tropical coastal waters.

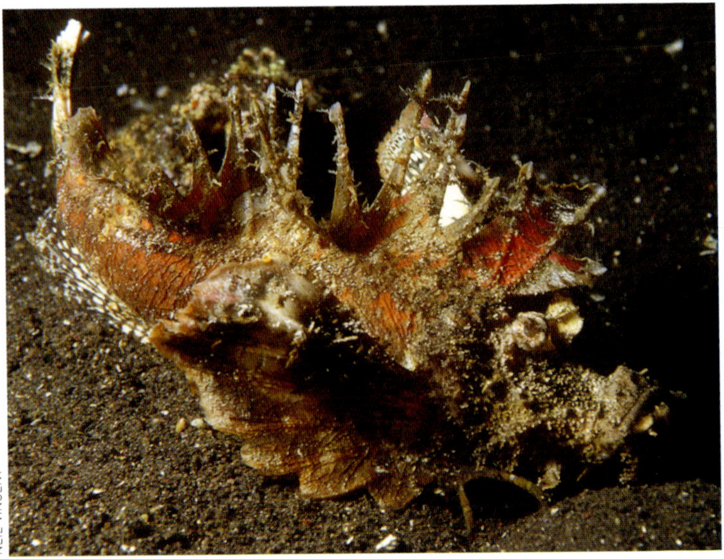

NEIL VINCENT

Symptoms **(First Aid — see page 54)**

Puncture wound 2–5mm in diameter. Immediate pain, increasing rapidly in intensity until it becomes excruciating. Pain lessens after some hours. Wound becomes swollen, hot, numb at centre but very tender at edges. Tissue around wound becomes red or bluish.

BUTTERFLY COD ★★★

(Red Fire Fish, Lion Fish, Zebra Fish, Coral Cod, Fire Cod, Turkey Fish, Tigerfish)

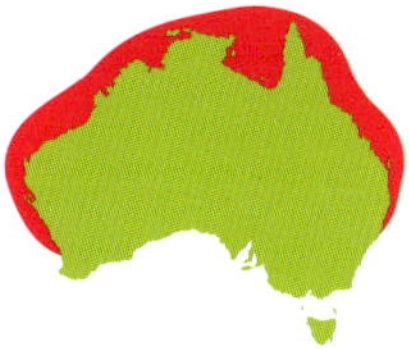

Up to 35cm long. Brightly coloured, with long feathery fins. Thirteen long spines along the back. If threatened these fish will erect their spines forward towards the threat. They have been known to jab at the hand of a diver reaching towards them. Found around reefs and rocks. Coastal temperate and tropical waters.

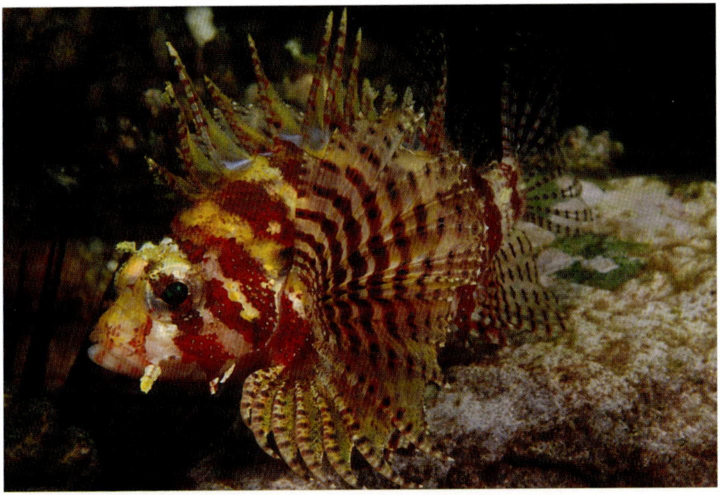

NEIL VINCENT

Symptoms (First Aid — see page 54)

Puncture wound a few millimetres in diameter. Immediate pain, increasing rapidly in intensity until it becomes excruciating. Pain lessens after some hours. Wound becomes swollen, hot, numb at centre but very tender at edges. Tissue around wound becomes red or bluish.

RED ROCK COD ★★★

(Mouth Almighty, Red Scorpion Cod)

Up to 35cm long. Mainly red and orange but will adopt colour of surrounding rocks. Twelve spines on back, many short, sharp spines on head. Large mouth.

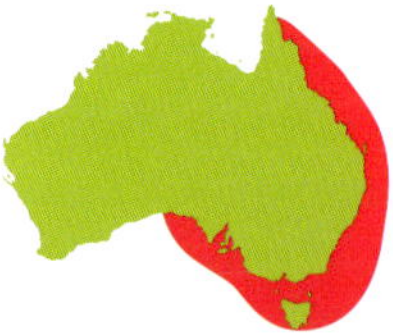

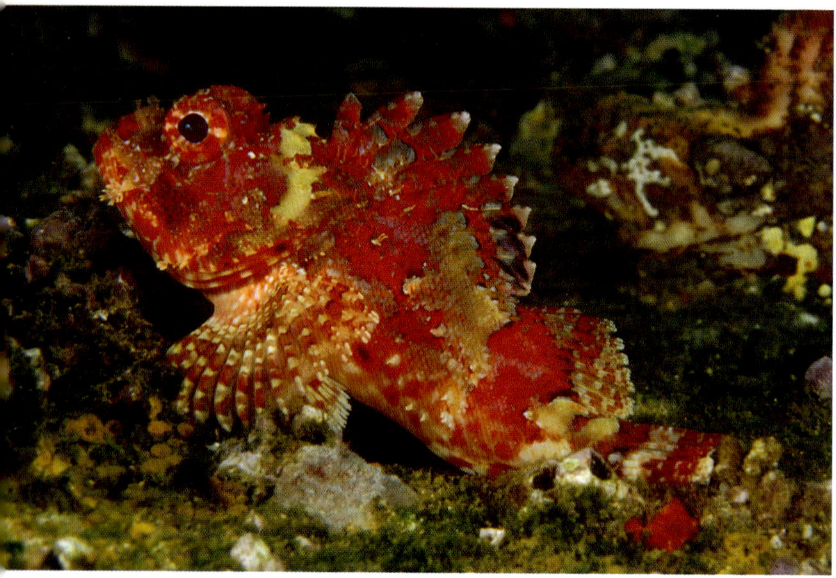

NEIL VINCENT

Symptoms (First Aid — see page 54)

Puncture wound. Immediate pain, increasing rapidly in intensity until it becomes excruciating. Pain lessens after some hours. Wound becomes swollen; surrounding tissue becomes red or bluish.

FORTESCUE ★★★

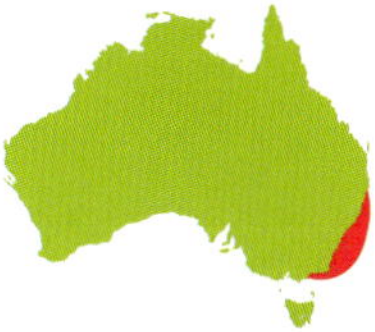

5–10cm long. Sixteen spines along the back. Pale coloured with darker bands. Slow moving. Normally found in harbours and estuaries.

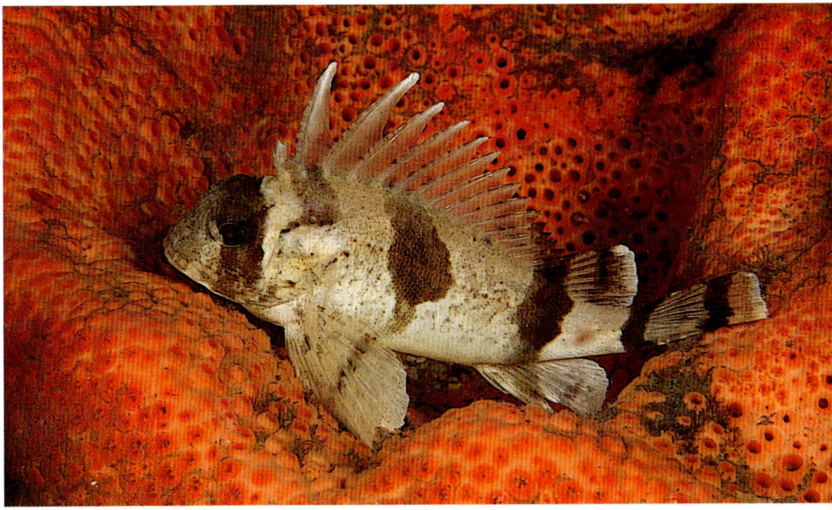

BECCA SAUNDERS

Symptoms (First Aid — see page 54)

Puncture wounds. Immediate pain, increasing rapidly in intensity until it becomes excruciating. Pain lessens to a dull ache after some hours. Tissue around wound becomes red or bluish.

FISH

BULLROUT ★★★

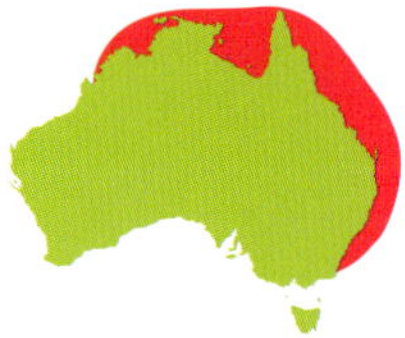

10–30cm long. Fifteen spines on the back. Brownish with black blotching. Rivers and estuaries; usually lies concealed in weed or reed beds. Will migrate up rivers and can be found well upriver away from the coast. May congregate below barriers such as dams and weirs.

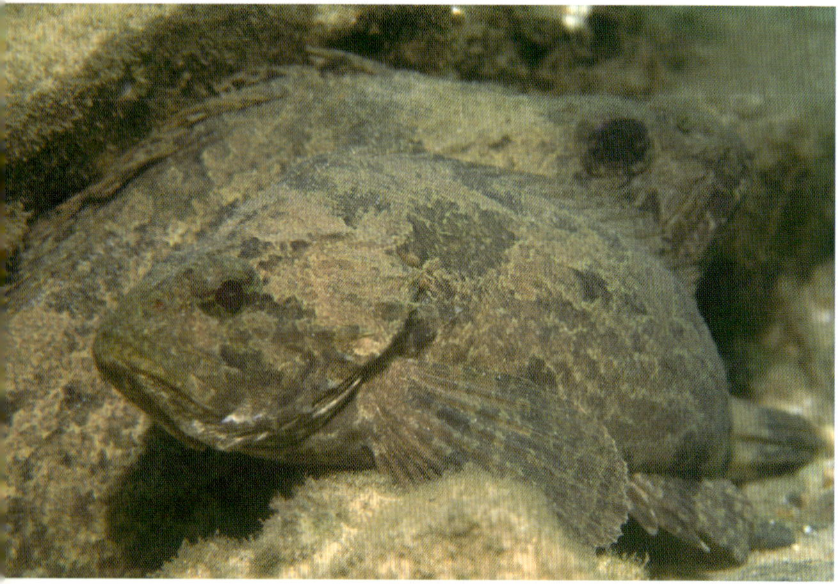

ERIK SCHLOGL

Symptoms (First Aid — see page 54)

Puncture wound 2–5mm in diameter. Immediate pain, increasing rapidly in intensity until it becomes excruciating. Pain lessens after some hours. Wound becomes numb; tissue around wound becomes red or bluish.

STARGAZER ★★★

15–75cm long. Cream to brown, with a square head, a vertical mouth with fringed lips and eyes on top of head. One shoulder spine behind the upper end of each gill opening. Buries itself in sand and mud.

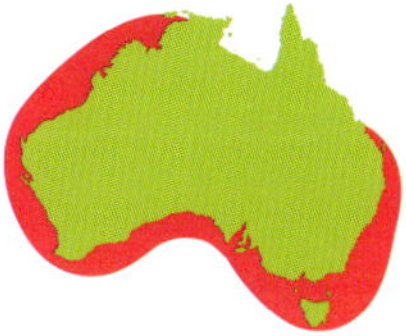

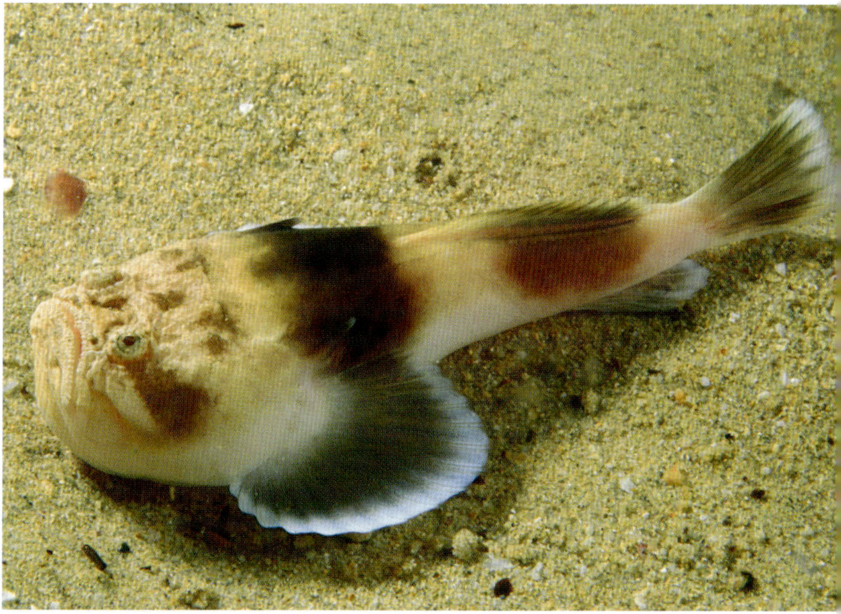

MARINETHEMES.COM/KELVIN AITKEN

Symptoms (First Aid — see page 54)

Puncture wound. Immediate pain, increasing rapidly in intensity. Pain lessens after some hours. Wound becomes numb; tissue around wound becomes red or bluish.

F

FISH

CAT FISH ★★★

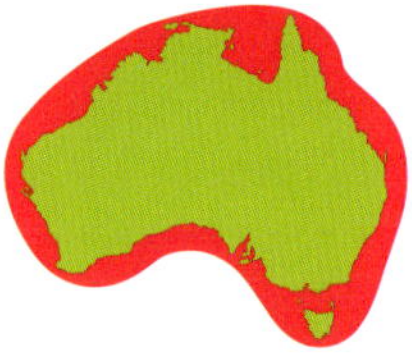

5cm–1m long. Several species occur in both fresh and salt water and in various colours and shapes. No scales. Barbels ('cat whiskers') around the mouth—these are not spines, but are used to detect food and to navigate. One very long spine on the back and one on each side of the body.

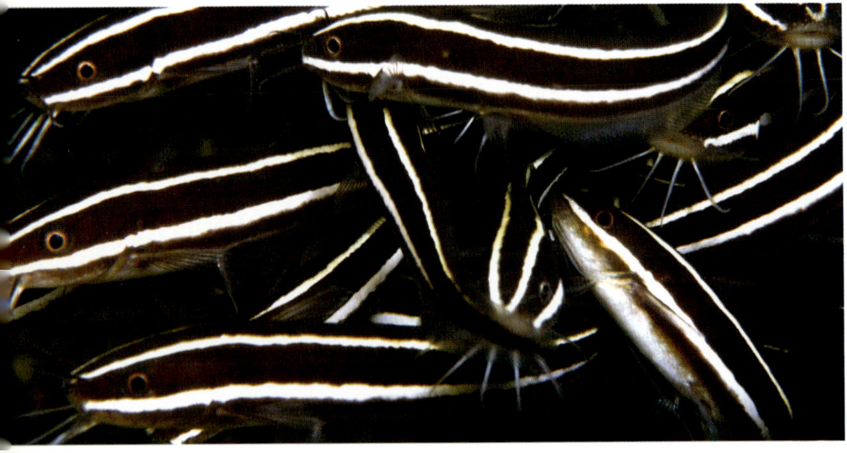

Symptoms (First Aid — see page 54)

Puncture wounds. Immediate pain, increasing rapidly in intensity. Pain lessens after some hours. Wound becomes swollen and numb; tissue around wound becomes red or bluish.

Additional First Aid

- Encourage bleeding from the wound—this reduces pain.

RABBITFISH ★★★

(Happy Moment)

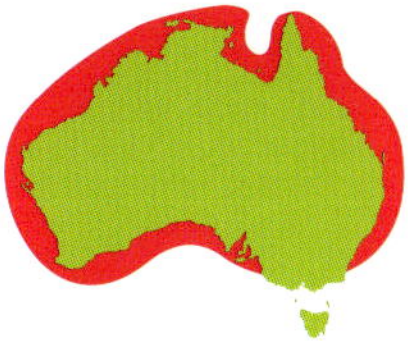

20–35cm long. Grey–green, yellow or blue with various markings. There are 13 spines on the back as well as another 11 underneath and on the sides.

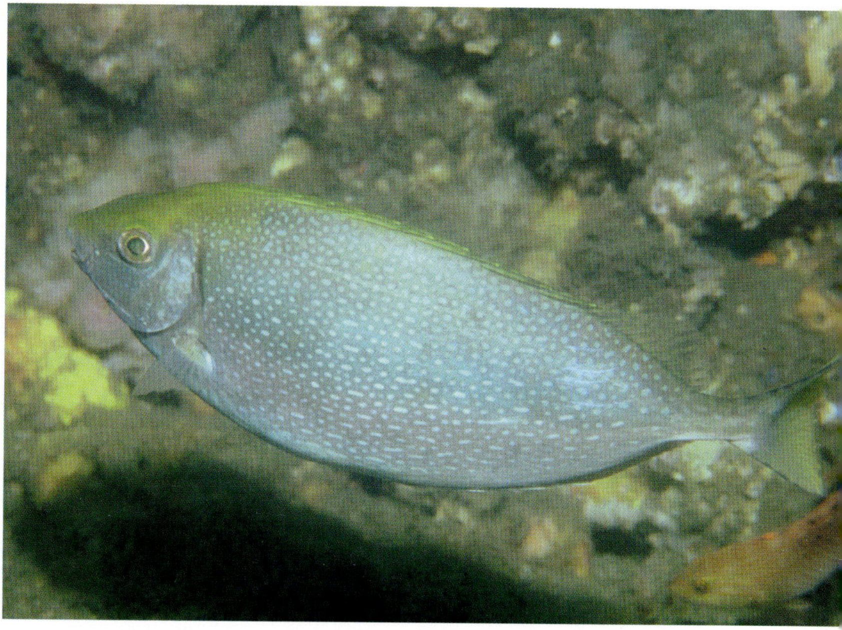

ERIK SCHLOGL

Symptoms (First Aid — see page 54)

A puncture wound or wounds, each 2–4mm in diameter. Immediate pain, increasing rapidly in intensity. Pain lessens after some hours. Wound becomes swollen and numb; tissue around wound becomes red or bluish.

OLD WIFE ★★★

(Zebra Fish)

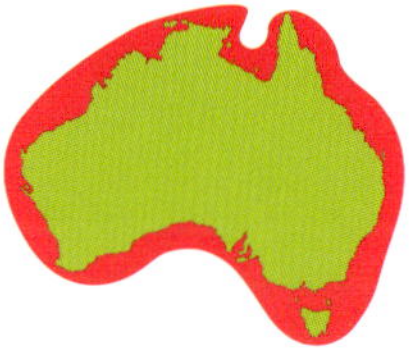

10–25cm long with zebra-like markings. The second spine on the back is far longer than the first. The name 'Old Wife' comes from its habit of grinding its teeth and making a grumbling sound when taken from the water. Common around wharfs and jetties as well as rocky reefs.

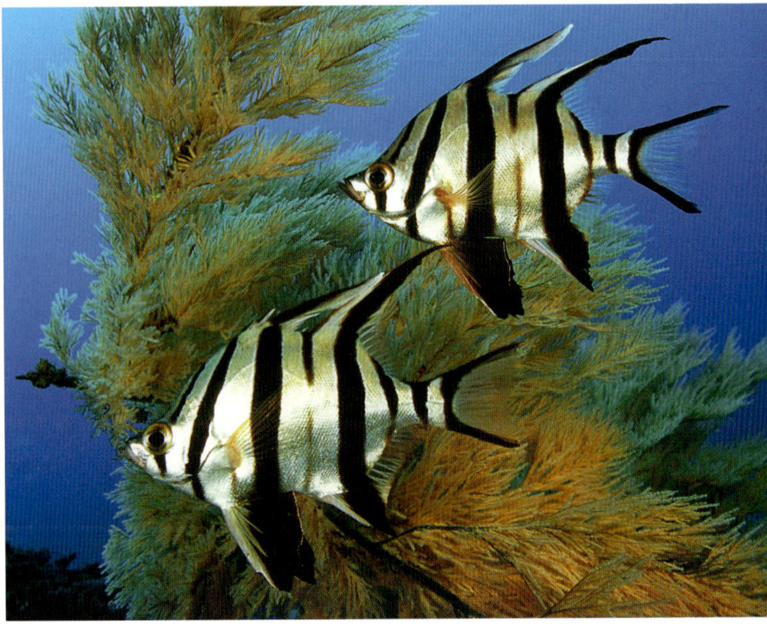

MARK SPENCER

Symptoms (First Aid — see page 54)

A sharp prick, followed by aching to severe pain. Wound becomes swollen; surrounding tissue becomes red or bluish.

FLEAS ★ F

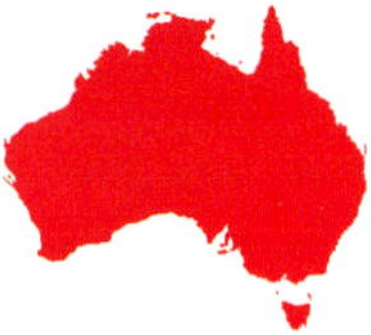

1.5–4mm long. Brown, wingless and flattened vertically, with long, jumping hind legs. Fleas are blood-sucking parasites that feed off the blood of people and animals. The most common fleas found in Australia are cat and dog fleas. With improved hygiene and living conditions, the human flea is not common now. Fleas can survive for some time without feeding and can become active upon picking up vibrations. This sometimes results in a 'flea plague' when an unoccupied house is reoccupied.

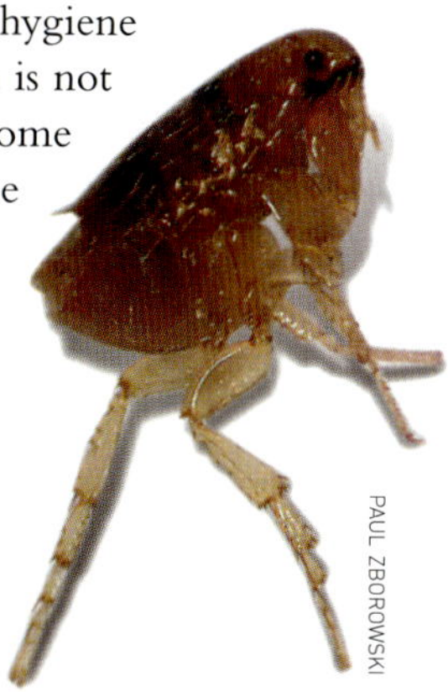

PAUL ZBOROWSKI

Symptoms

Lower legs and feet are common bite sites. Bites are very itchy with a red lump. Scratching the bites can cause infections.

First Aid

- Do not scratch the bites.
- Wash with soap and water.
- Apply ice pack/cold compress to reduce any swelling.
- Apply calamine lotion or an anaesthetic cream to help reduce the itching.
- If infection develops or victim has intense itching, consult a doctor.

F FLIES ★

HOUSE FLIES and blowflies are all well-known nuisances. Because of their attraction to garbage, excrement and carrion, they often spread dangerous bacteria and viruses. The bushfly is attracted to people's faces as it seeks moisture from sweat and eyes. Several types of fly do bite. These flies bite through the skin to feed on blood.

MARCH FLY

(Green Head)

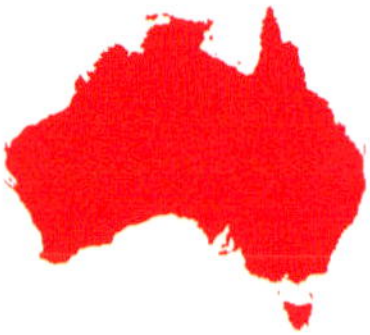

5–25mm long. Savage biters, but quite slow moving and easy to swat. They hover as they prepare to get blood. Large eyes are often green. Only breeding females bite to feed on blood. Males take pollen or nectar.

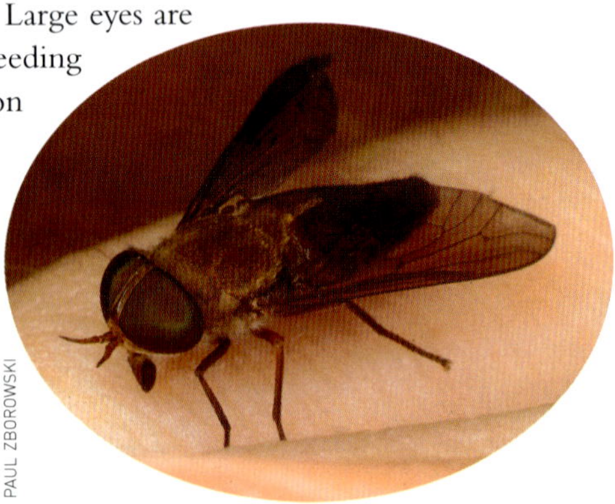

PAUL ZBOROWSKI

Symptoms

Sharp sting. Sometimes itching.

First Aid

- Apply ice pack or local anaesthetic cream if necessary.

SANDFLY

(Biting Midge, No-see-um)

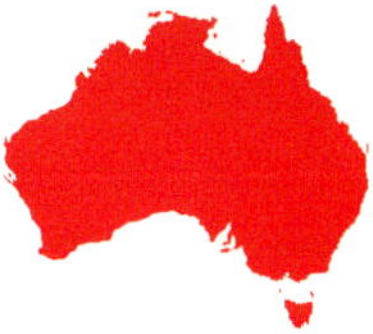

1–4mm long, with short legs. Dark with mottled wings that fold over abdomen when fly is resting. Sometimes occur in large hordes, making them a serious pest. Usually near water.

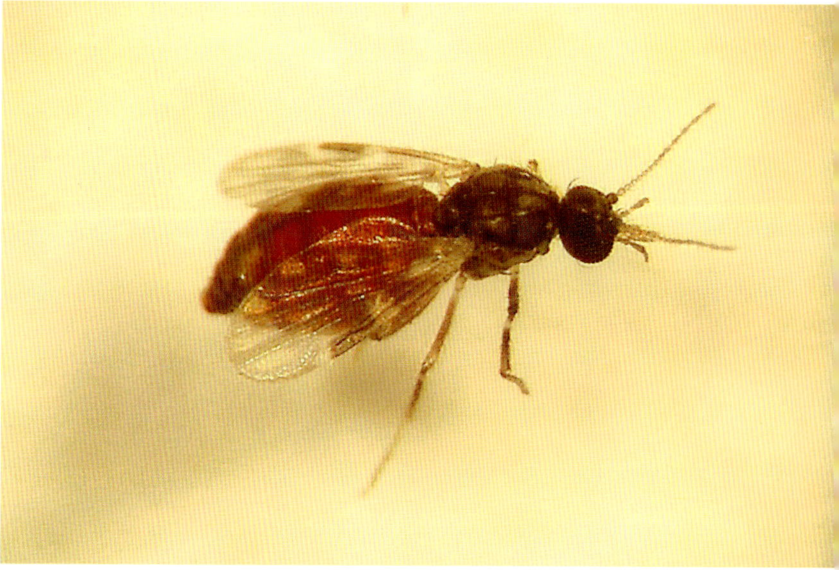

PAUL ZBOROWSKI

Symptoms

Itchiness and swelling.

First Aid

- Apply ice pack/cold compress to reduce swelling.
- Apply calamine lotion to reduce itchiness.

F FROGS ★★★

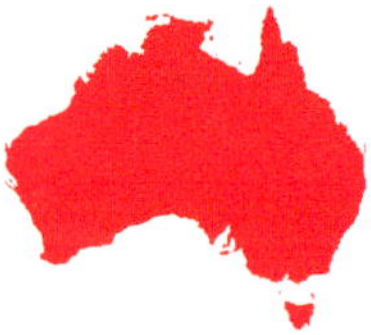

THERE ARE over 200 species of frogs in Australia and they come in all sizes, shapes and colours. Generally, they are completely harmless, but the skin of some species of frogs contains toxic substances. Kissing frogs is a practice to be discouraged, particularly among children. While the poison arrow frogs of Central and South America are well known for their poisonous skin secretions, some of which can kill within seconds, the toxic nature of Australian frog skin secretions is not well known, nor has much research been done. Always wash your hands after handling a frog.

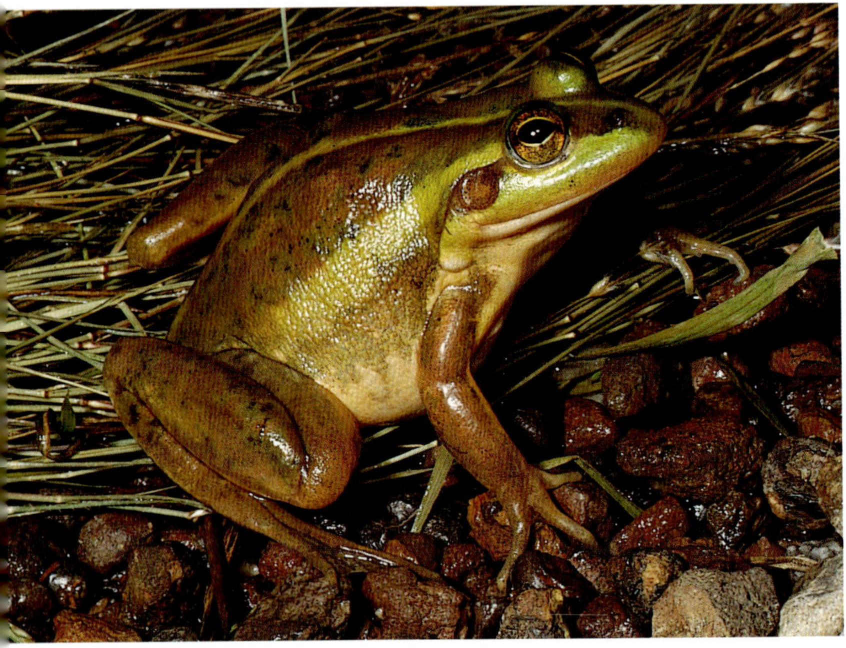

ROB VALENTIC

Dahl's Frog

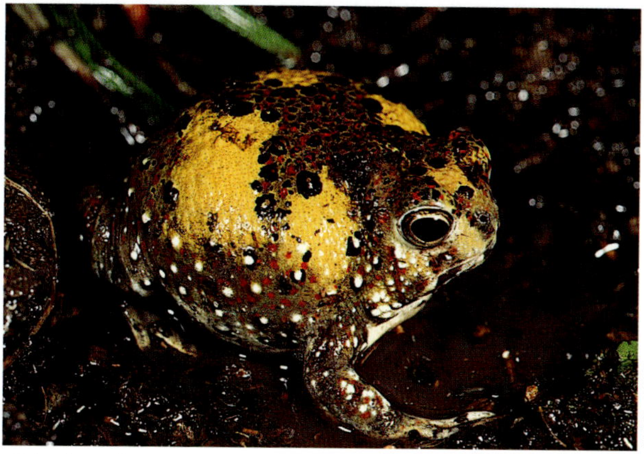

Holy Cross Frog

Symptoms

If skin secretion comes into contact with eyes
Intense burning sensation and irritation of eye.

If skin secretion comes into contact with mouth
Swollen lips, completely dry lips and mouth. Constriction of respiratory tract and difficulty breathing. Slowing down of heart rate lasting about 30 minutes. (Symptoms are based on two recorded cases in Australia.)

First Aid

Eyes
- Bathe eyes with water until symptoms are relieved.

Mouth
- Wash mouth with water.
- Seek medical aid.
- Have victim lie down and rest.

J JELLYFISH

As JELLYFISH look nothing like fish, the name jellies is now often used instead. Jellyfish include sea jellies, box jellies and bluebottles, the latter of which are not jellyfish but a floating colony of individual organisms. Some jellyfish are deadly. Do not touch them—even the tentacles of dead jellyfish can sting.

BLUEBOTTLE ★★

(Portuguese Man-o'-war)

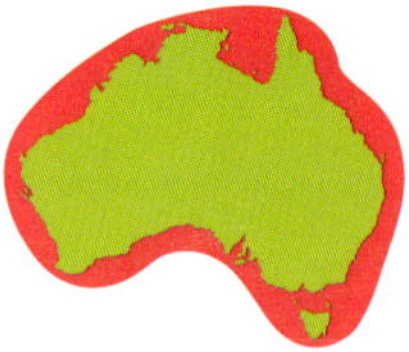

The blue float (up to 10cm long) allows the Bluebottle to stay on top of the water but also puts it at the mercy of the wind. The tentacles hanging underneath can trail for 3m. Found in shallow water or blown onto beaches.

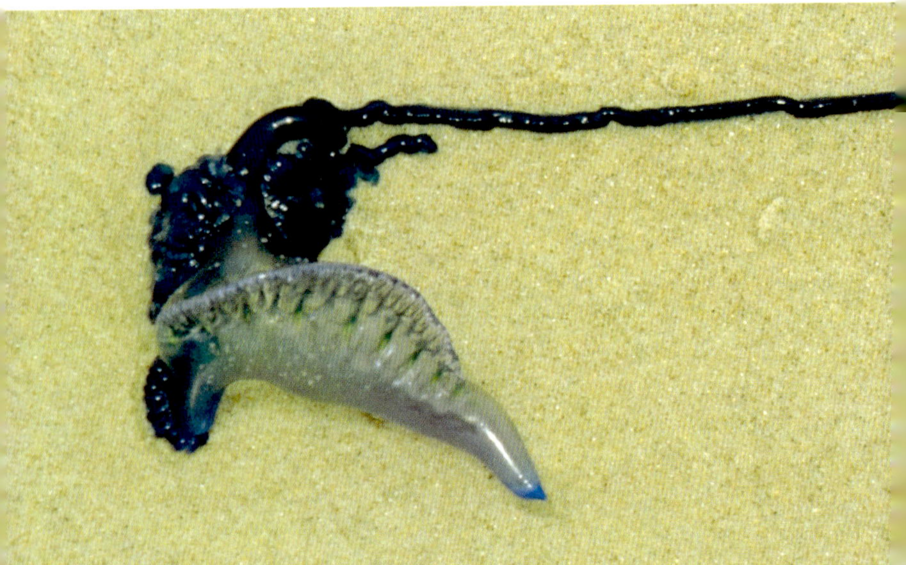

Symptoms

Injury usually a single long whip-like strip of inflamed skin. Sharp, severe pain can last a few hours. There may be sweating, itching and nausea.

First Aid

- Remove victim from water.
- Remove adhering tentacles gently, with tweezers. Do not touch tentacles.
- Apply hot water to relieve pain. Take care not to scald victim.
- If reaction is severe, seek medical aid.
- Do not apply vinegar as this may cause more venom to be injected.

GEOFF SWAN

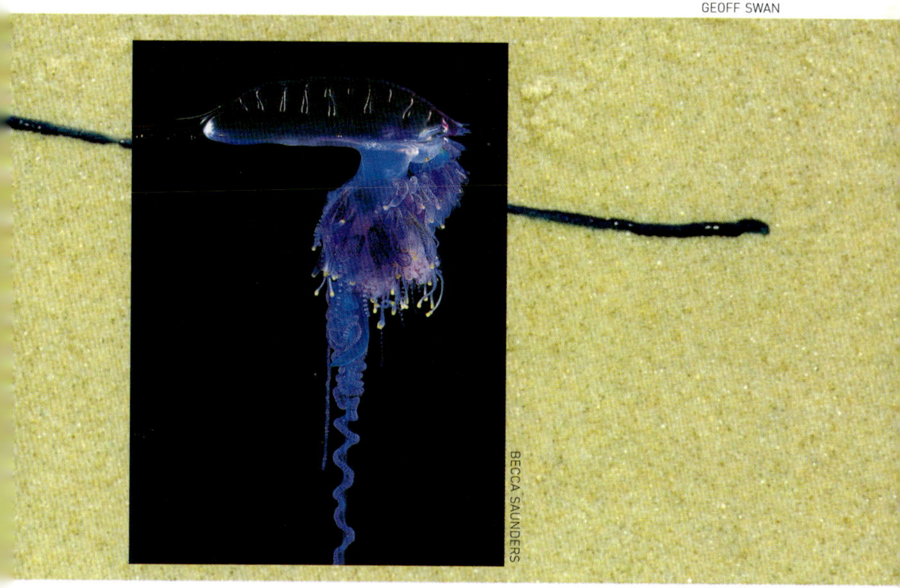

BECCA SAUNDERS

J JELLYFISH

BOX JELLYFISH ★★★★

(Sea Wasp, Indringa, Fire Medusa, Chironex, Flecker's Box Jelly)

Almost transparent—difficult to see in the water. Square-shaped body can be 30cm across. Multiple tentacles are suspended from the four corners and can be 3m long. Around the northern coast during the warmer months (October–April).

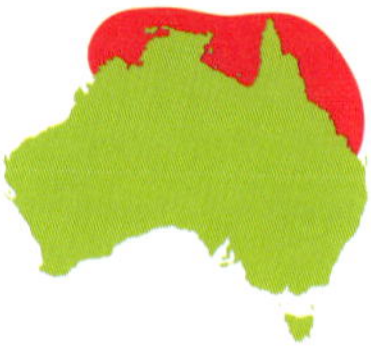

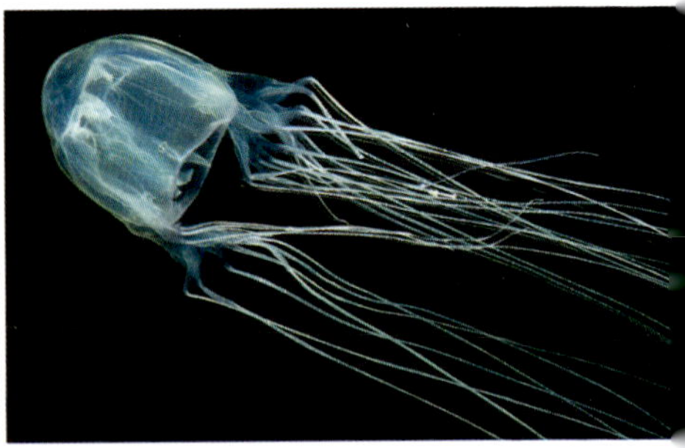

MARIINETHEMES.COM/KELVIN AITKEN

Symptoms

Injury shows as swollen lines of purple or dark brown. In severe cases the skin can be permanently scarred or discoloured. Immediate agonising pain that may cause incoherence. Loss of consciousness, cessation of breathing and death.

First Aid

- Remove victim from water and prevent them from rubbing the stung area.
- Apply copious amounts of household vinegar to the tentacles for at least 30 seconds. This stops more venom being discharged from the tentacles.
- Apply pressure-immobilisation bandage (see page 15) over stung area if this is on a limb. Apply bandage above stung area if it has not been washed with vinegar.
- If necessary commence EAR or CPR (see pages 11–12).
- Take victim to hospital urgently. Antivenom is available.

IRUKANDJI ★★★

1–2cm long. Transparent box jelly with four tentacles up to 1m long. Coastal waters. Ocean-going, but carried to beaches by suitable winds or currents. Most stings occur during the summer months in shallow water but divers in deeper water have also been stung.

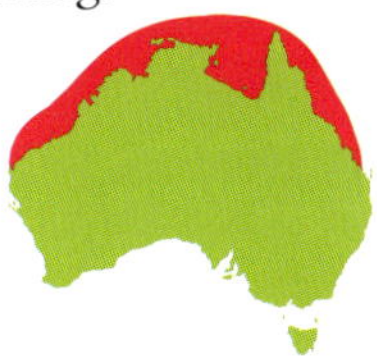

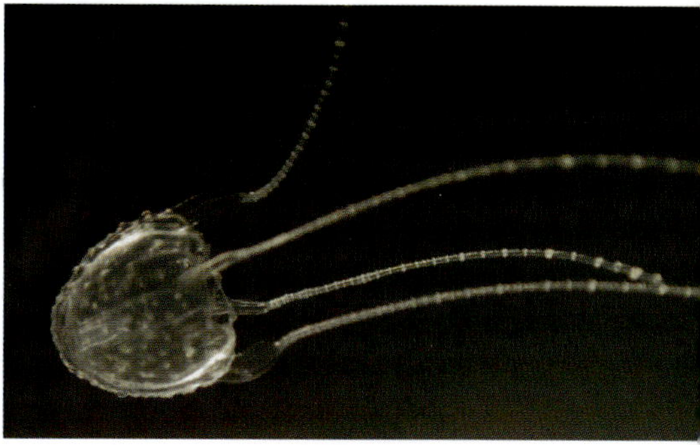

JAMIE SEYMOUR

Symptoms

Jelly is not usually seen by the swimmer. Initial contact is a minor sting that leaves a red mark on the skin. The main symptoms may not occur for 10–60 minutes, and are not always associated with the earlier sting. There may be a low backache which develops into severe abdominal pain, and cramps in the limbs, abdomen and chest, which often come in waves. These have been confused with a gastric condition or heart attack. Profuse sweating, headaches and vomiting may also occur.

First Aid

- Remove victim from water, keep warm and comfortable and reassure.
- Apply an ice pack to the stung area.
- Check breathing and pulse. If necessary commence EAR or CPR (see pages 11–12).
- Seek medical aid immediately.

J JELLYFISH

JIMBLE ★★★

(Lantern Medusa)

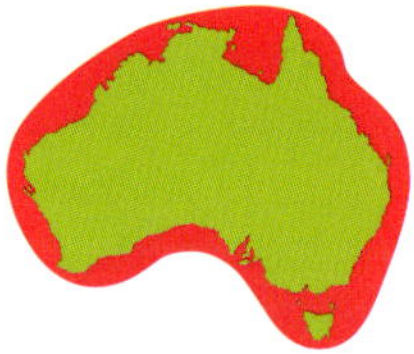

About 1cm across. Box-shaped, transparent body with four 5cm mauve tentacles, one at each corner. Usually occur in swarms. Coastal areas.

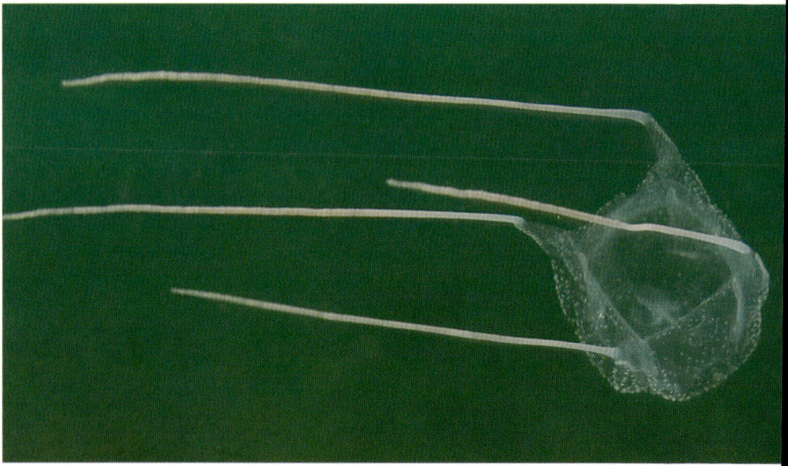

NEIL VINCENT

Symptoms

Painful sting that may last up to two hours, with swelling and redness.

First Aid

- Remove victim from water.
- Gently remove tentacles from skin with tweezers.
- Apply ice pack/cold compress or local anaesthetic cream to help reduce pain.
- Seek medical aid if symptoms persist.

HAIRY STINGER ★★★

(Sea Blubber, Sea Nettle, Hairy Jelly, Lion's Mane, Cyanea)

Flattened red, pink or yellow body up to 1m across with eight clusters of 1–10m long tentacles. Coastal waters.

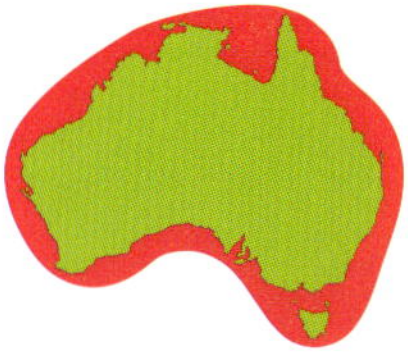

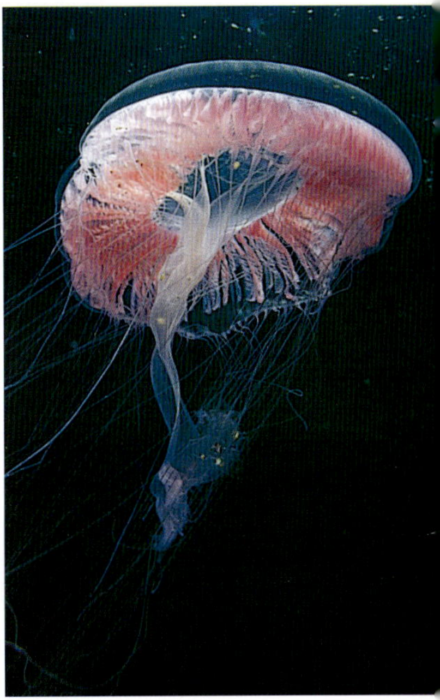

MARK SPENCER

Symptoms

Painful sting that may last up to two hours with swelling and redness. Sweating, nausea and vomiting may occur within minutes or after several hours. There can also be abdominal pains and muscle cramps.

First Aid

- Remove victim from water.
- Gently remove tentacles with tweezers.
- Apply local anaesthetic cream or ice pack/cold compress.
- If reaction is severe, seek medical aid.

L LEECHES ★

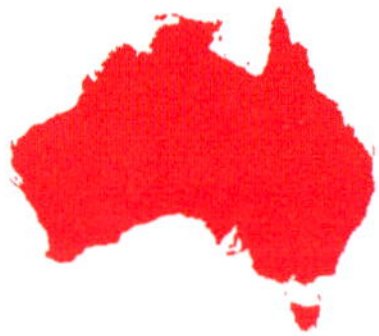

20–85mm long. Slimy black or brown. Some have a yellow or orange stripe along the body. They move with a quite distinct looping action that involves alternately attaching their front and back suckers to the surface. Leeches have had a long history in medicine and at one time were used to treat just about every known disease and ailment. Moist forested areas, freshwater ponds and other water bodies.

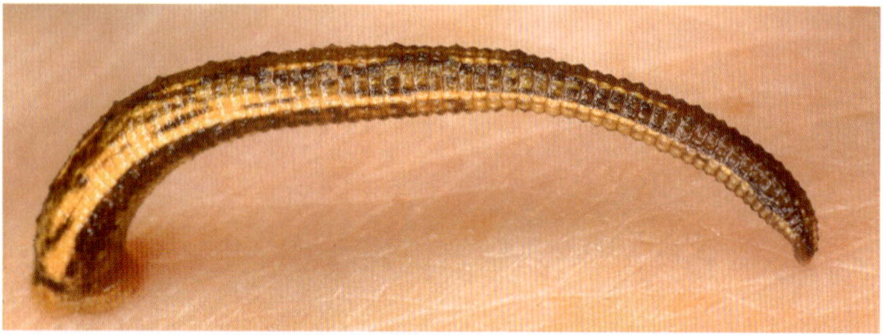

PAUL ZBOROWSKI

Symptoms

The first indication is probably a bleeding wound on the foot or leg. Leeches inject an anti-clotting chemical at the bite, causing bleeding to continue after the leech has dropped off. Leech bites will often itch for days.

First Aid

- If the leech is still attached, do not pull it off as this could cause a nasty wound. To make it let go sprinkle some salt on it, or apply heat in the form of a cigarette or lighted match.
- Once the leech has been removed, let the wound bleed for a minute or so then wash and apply calamine lotion.
- Cover the wound with a bandaid.

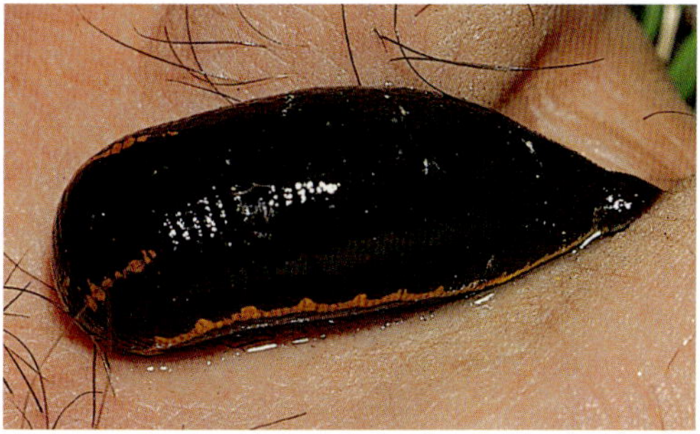

PETER MARSACK/LT

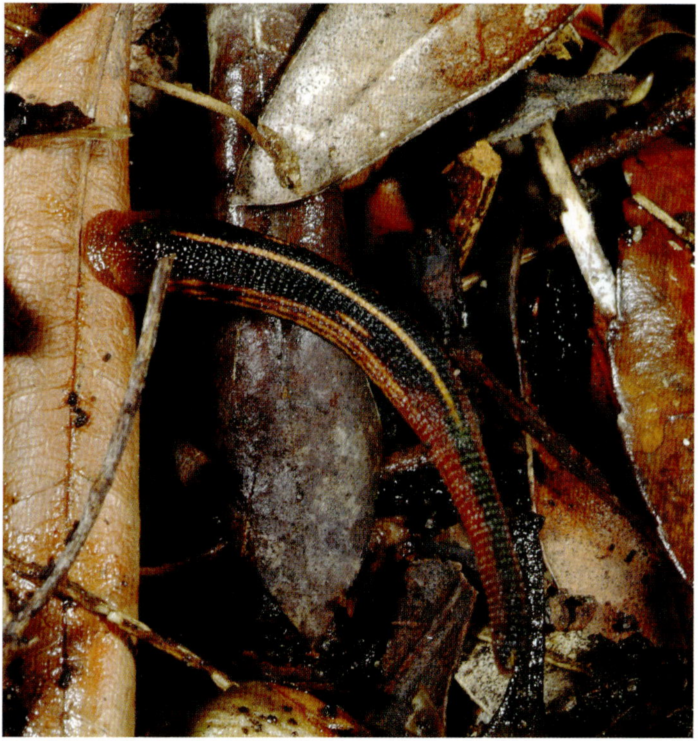

GEOFF SWAN

L LICE ★

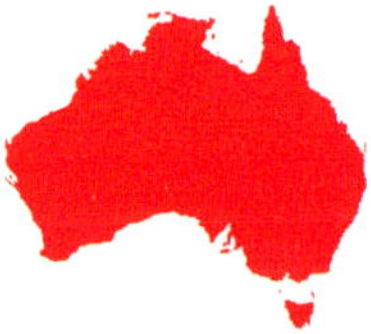

Lice are blood-sucking parasites that are often host specific. Those of concern to people are the Head Louse, the Body Louse and the Pubic Louse (also known as the Crab Louse). Not only are they found exclusively on humans, but Head Lice can only survive on the scalp, while Body Lice cannot live on the head. Body Lice are uncommon in Australia.

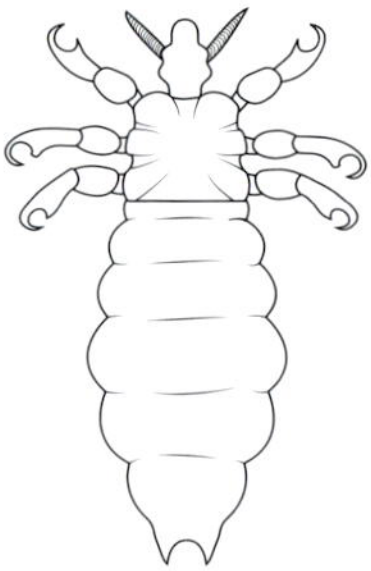

HEAD LICE

2.5–3.5mm long. Light brown, flattened body, small antennae and well-developed eyes. Live only in human hair, where they suck blood from the scalp. White lice eggs, known as nits, are laid at the base of a strand of hair.

Symptoms

Head lice are contagious and a nuisance but are not responsible for the spread of any infectious disease-carrying organisms. Irritation and itching of the scalp with resultant scratching are usually the first sign of an infestation. Finding eggs (nits) firmly attached to strands of hair is a common way of identifying an infestation.

First Aid

- Treat victim immediately with one of the wide range of preparations obtainable from a chemist.
- Treat all close contacts as well.
- Wash all towels and bed linen.
- Repeat treatment after seven days.
- Use a lice comb to remove nits.

PUBIC LICE

(Crab Lice, Crabs)

1.25–2mm long, with a crab-like appearance. Grey with an oval body and very large second and third pairs of legs. Usually occur in pubic hair, but sometimes found in other coarse hair on the body such as beard, armpits and eyebrows. Lice eggs (nits) are laid on strands of hair.

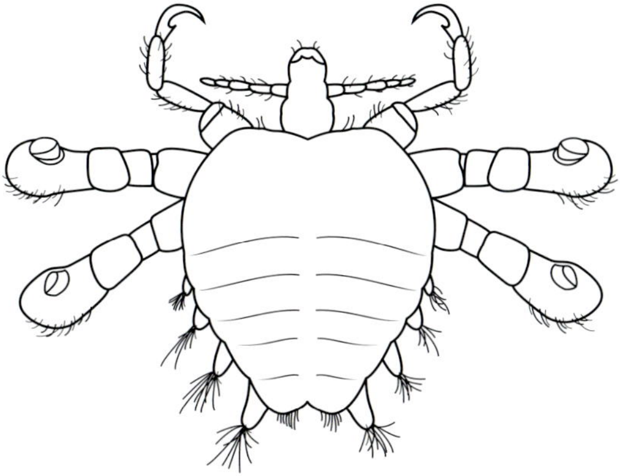

Symptoms

These lice are not known for the spread of any infectious disease-carrying organisms in Australia. At each bite site there is swelling and a red pimple. Intense itching.

First Aid

- Treat victim immediately with one of the wide range of preparations obtainable from a chemist.
- Treat all close contacts and family as well.
- Wash underwear and bed clothes of victim in hot water and tumble dry.

L LIZARDS ★–★★★

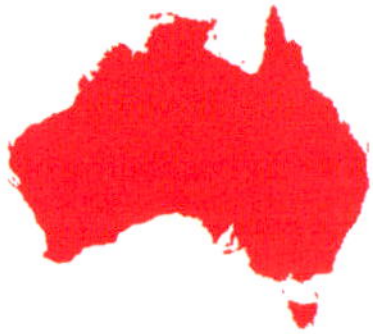

Any lizard will bite if it feels threatened. Many, like the blue-tongues, have blunt peg-like teeth, and while a bite can be painful, it will not break the skin. Others have sharp teeth and can bite through to the bone, causing severe lacerations and infection. None is venomous. Avoid handling and warn children not to approach too close. Large lizards can inflict painful bites and, in the case of goannas, these can be dangerous.

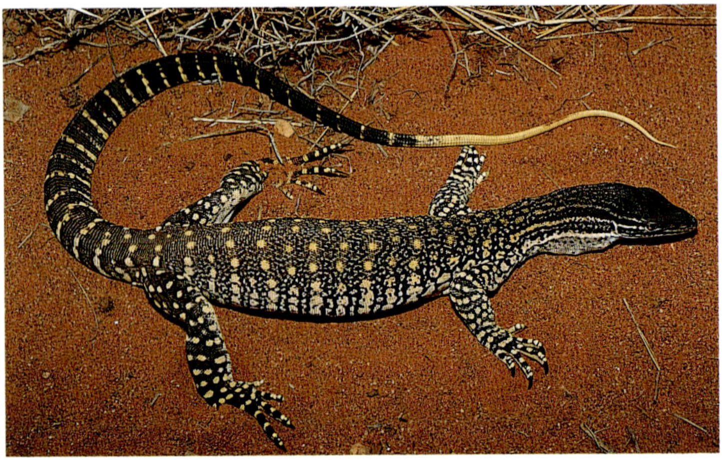

GEOFF SWAN

Sand Goanna

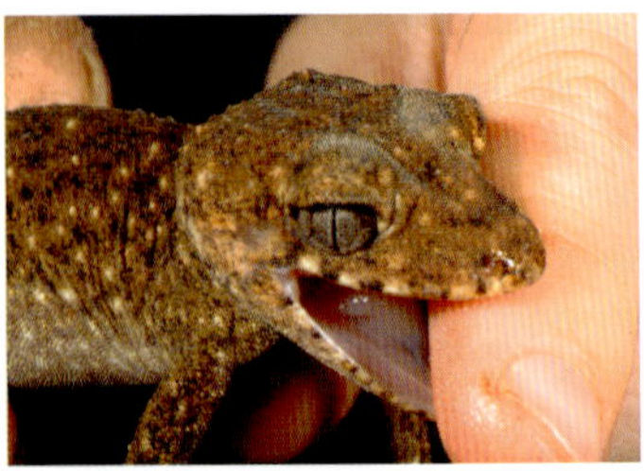

GEOFF SWAN

Gecko bites are harmless.

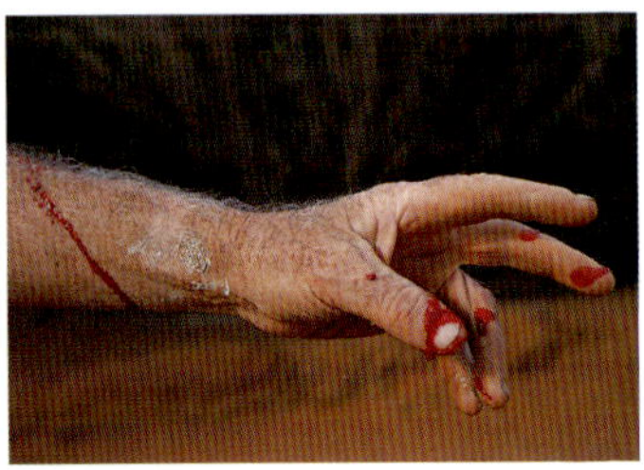

GEOFF SWAN

Goanna bite

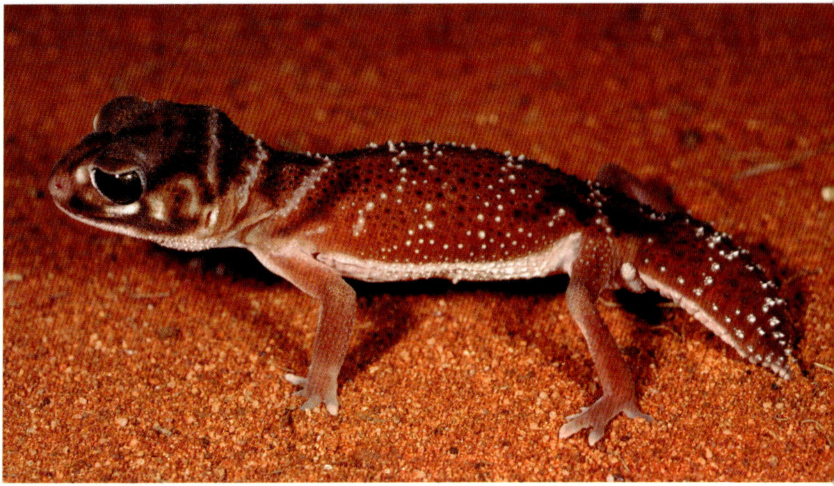
GEOFF SWAN

Knob-tailed Gecko

Symptoms

Depending upon the type and size of lizard there may be only a row of teeth marks, some grazes, small puncture wounds with bleeding, or deep puncture wounds or lacerations and copious bleeding.

First Aid

- If the lizard is still hanging on, place it on the ground and do not restrain or touch it. This will often be sufficient to induce it to release its grip.
- Control bleeding if necessary (see page 14).
- Wash wounds with water and antiseptic.
- If wounds are severe, seek medical aid.
- Such wounds may become infected; if necessary treat with antibiotics.

M MITES

MITES ARE very small, most being only just visible to the naked eye, while some are microscopic. They suck liquid food from their prey. Many feed on plants, some feed on invertebrates, others are parasites of people and animals.

DUST MITES ★★

0.5mm long. Whitish. Difficult to see without magnification. Live in the fine layer of dust that settles in a house, concentrating in carpets, beds and lounge furniture. Favour high humidity and constant warm temperatures.

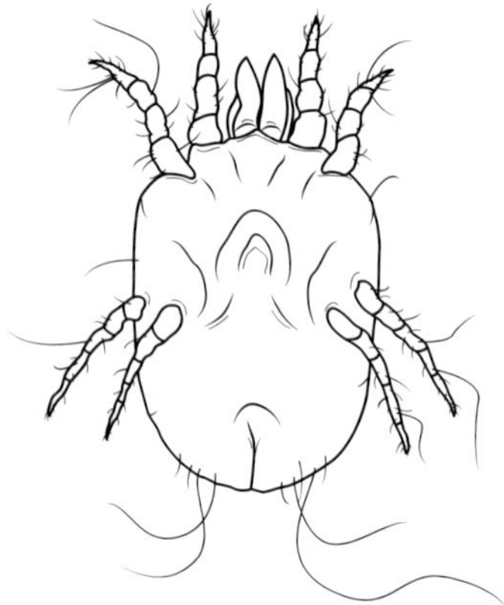

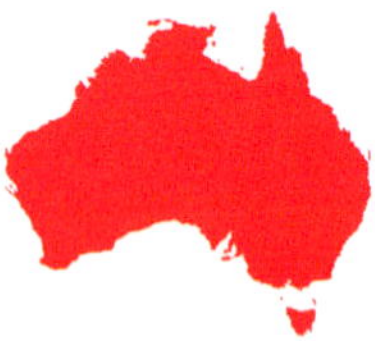

Symptoms

Dust mites do not transmit any disease-causing pathogens. They do not bite or sting, but constant contact with them can cause allergic conditions such as asthma and eczema.

First Aid

- Consult your doctor.
- Reduce mite populations by regular, thorough vacuuming, frequent washing of bedding and curtains, and removal of carpets.

BIRD MITES ★

0.5mm long. Semi-transparent or reddish black. Only just visible to the naked eye. Bird mites infest nests in huge numbers. When nests are abandoned, mites leave to find new bird hosts. They will 'test bite' humans but cannot survive on human blood.

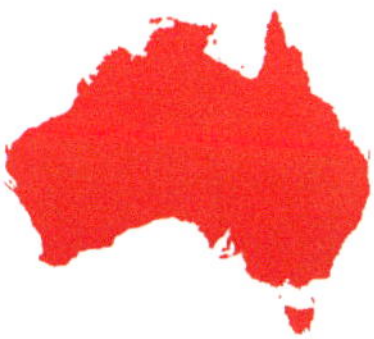

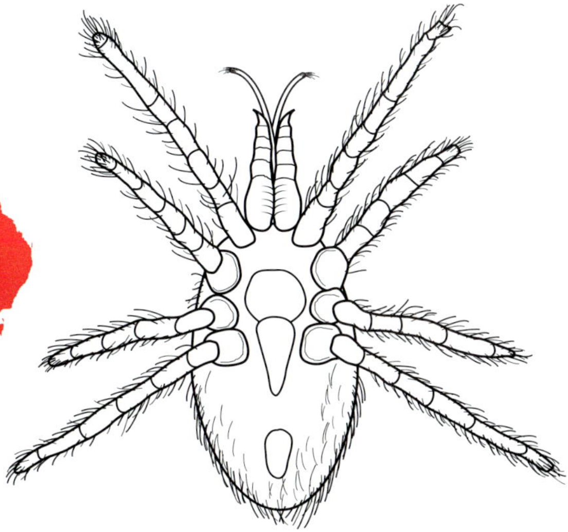

Symptoms

Intense itching, rashes. Scratching bites can cause infections.

First Aid

- Apply an anti-itch medication such as calamine lotion to relieve the irritation.
- Locate and remove source of infestation (nests in gutters, roofs etc.).

M

MITES

SCABIES MITES ★★

0.2–0.4mm long. Oval, light-coloured parasitic mites that live under human skin.

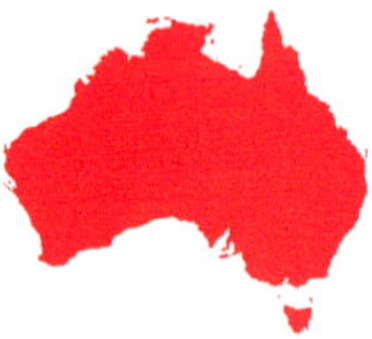

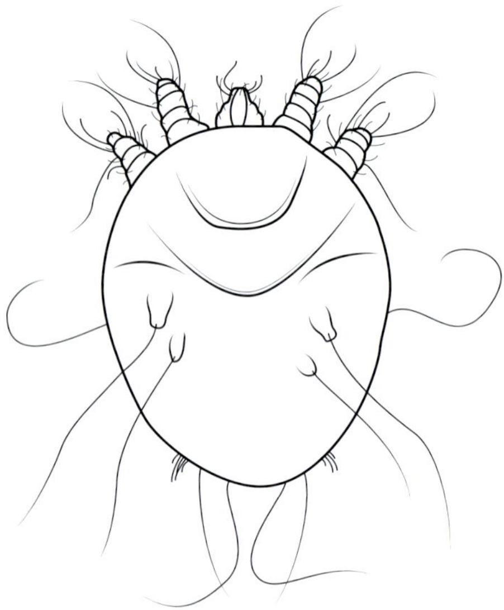

Symptoms

Often burrow into the skin on the hands, between the fingers, and on wrists and elbows. On the surface the tunnels look like grey pencil marks. Severe itching all over the body, often at night. Rashes may develop. Scratching can cause infections.

First Aid

- Apply a chemical preparation available from a chemist.
- Wash bed linen and underwear in hot water and then tumble dry.

CHIGGERS ★★★

The larvae of a mite that occurs in various regions of the Pacific and Asia. The mite itself does not bite humans but the larvae feed on skin tissue and attach themselves, burrowing beneath the skin. Adults are 1–2mm long, red–brown, with a velvety appearance. Larvae are about 0.15mm long and not visible to the naked eye.

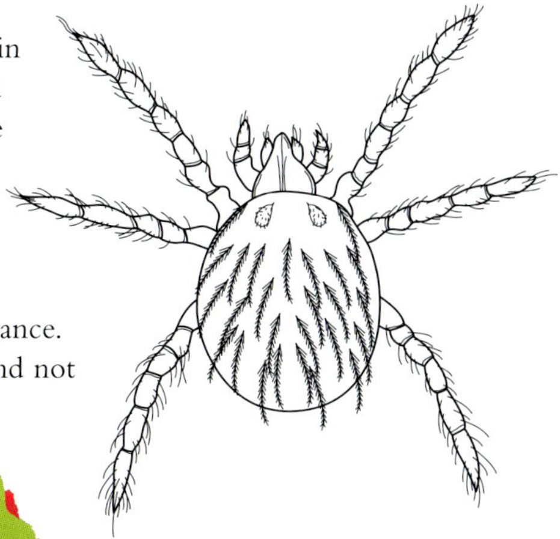

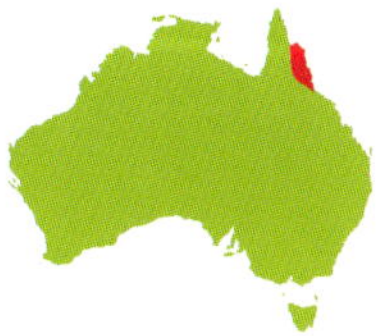

Symptoms

Usually bites are around the ankles or waist. Severe itching, inflammation and slight swelling, red in the centre, fills with fluid and bursts leaving a black scab.

Chigger bites can result in scrub typhus. Symptoms include chills, fever, severe headache, a red spotted rash on the body and tender lymph glands. Incubation period 10–12 days.

First Aid

- Apply local anaesthetic cream to relieve itching.
- If scrub typhus symptoms appear, seek immediate medical aid.

M MOSQUITOES

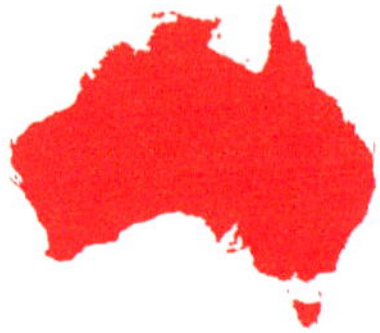

4–6mm long. Over 300 species of small, fragile blood-sucking insects with six long, delicate legs and a projecting proboscis that contains the long piercing and sucking mouthparts.

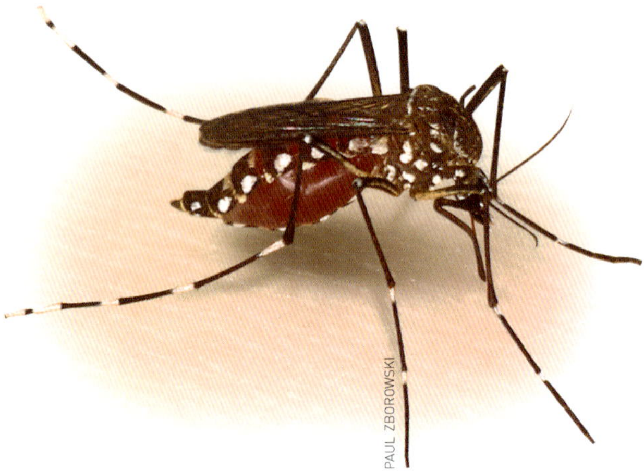

Symptoms

Swelling, redness and itching at the bite site caused by an allergic reaction to the saliva discharged by the mosquito during its probing into the skin. Scratching can cause infection.

First Aid

- Ice pack/cold compress can help reduce swelling and pain.
- Antihistamines may help relieve itchiness.

Mosquito-borne Diseases in Australia

Mosquitoes transmit many diseases through human and animal populations, but only a few are of concern. These are the species that carry Dengue fever, Australian encephalitis, Ross River fever and Malaria.

★★★★ **Malaria** is no longer endemic in Australia, but cases occur in travellers infected elsewhere. Usually causes severe fever, but fatal complications can occur. Seek medical aid.

★★★ **Dengue virus** is usually imported into Australia by travellers infected elsewhere. Transmitted by one species of mosquito in Australia that occurs in Qld, but historically occurred in NSW, WA and the NT. Causes fever, headaches and muscle and joint pains. Mainly affects older children and adults, lasting about four to seven days. More severe form with internal bleeding occurs more frequently in young children. Seek medical aid.

★★★ **Ross River and Barmah Forest viruses** are active Australia-wide. They cause rashes with fevers, arthritis affecting ankles, knees, fingers and wrists mainly, although other joints may be affected. In mild cases recovery is usually less than one month, but in severe cases it can persist for many months to years. Seek medical aid.

★★★★ **Australian encephalitis (Murray Valley encephalitis, Kunjin virus)** occurs in northern and south-eastern Australia. Cases vary from mild to fatal. The viruses cause encephalitis (inflammation of the brain). Fever, often with anorexia and headache. Vomiting, nausea, diarrhoea and dizziness may also be experienced. Brain dysfunction may be experienced after a few days with lethargy, irritability, drowsiness, confusion, convulsions and fits. Coma and death can ensue. Seek medical aid.

M MUSHROOMS & TOADSTOOLS ★★★

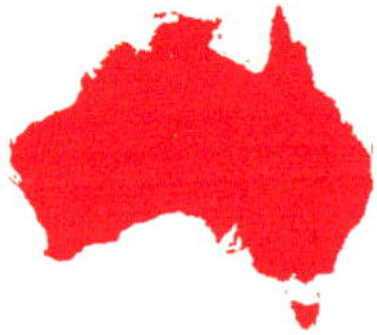

THERE IS no simple, general guide to determine if a mushroom is edible or poisonous. Even if it is identified using one of the guides available, there may be no recorded information on its edibility. Sampling wild fungi is risky and not advisable.

Most mushrooms are not poisonous but are too small, too rare, or too unpalatable to eat. Cooking poisonous mushrooms will not make them harmless. The test that a mushroom is safe if it peels is worthless. So too is the test that if cooking mushrooms tarnish a silver spoon, the mushroom is poisonous.

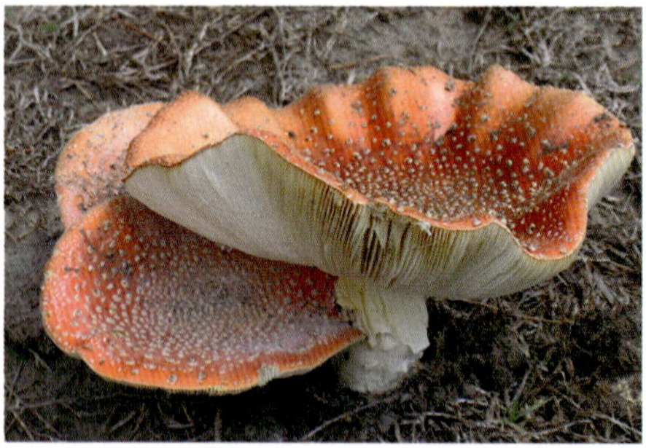

SANDY JACKA

Fly Agaric

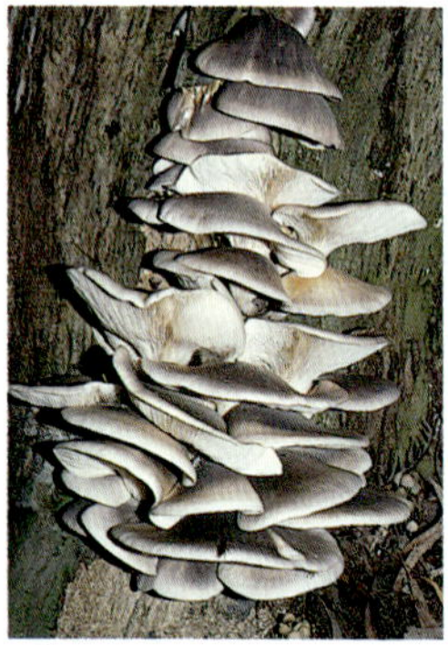

DENISE GREIG

Ghost Fungus

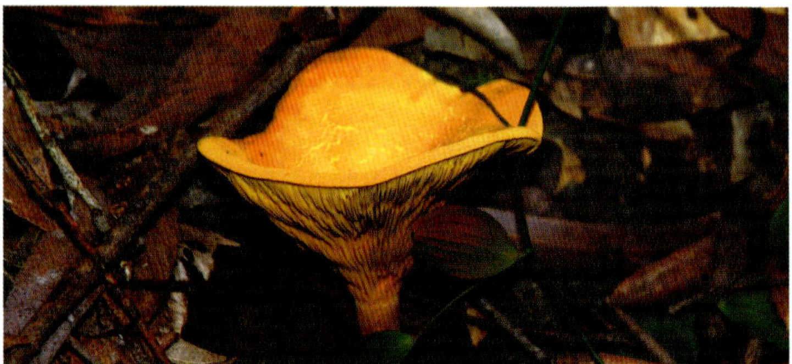

GEOFF SWAN

Funnel Pax

MUSHROOMS & TOADSTOOLS

1–100cm across cap depending upon species. Cap may be flat, curved or funnel shaped, and can come in all colours, as do gills underneath cap. From suburban lawns and gardens to pine forests and bushland.

The definitions of mushroom and toadstool, both of which are fungi, are imprecise. Mushroom is sometimes used to denote the edible fungi, while toadstool has been applied to the poisonous species. This is not correct and seems to have come about because most fungi do not have common names.

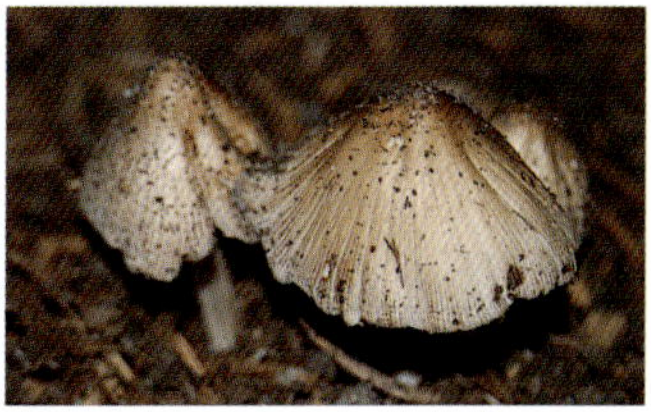

GEOFF SWAN

Ink Cap

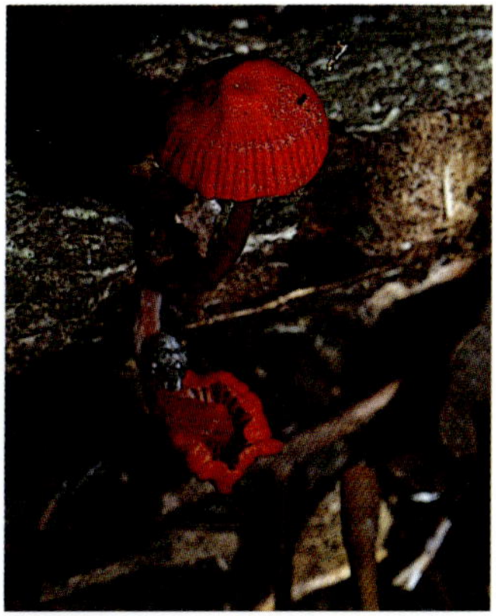

DENISE GREIG

Waxy Gills

Symptoms

Vomiting and diarrhoea may occur from half an hour to several hours after eating. There may be sweating, shivering, abdominal pains, or severe burning or numbness of the mouth.

First Aid

- Reassure the victim.
- Contact the Poisons Information Centre for advice (page 7).
- Seek medical aid.

P PLATYPUS ★★

40–60cm long. Fur-covered with webbed feet and a flexible duck-like bill. Female lays eggs and suckles her young on milk, which is secreted through pores on the belly and not through teats. Male platypuses are unique among mammals in being venomous. A sharp hollow spur on the inside of each hind leg is attached to a venom gland. Wounds only occur if the animal is handled. Permanent waterways.

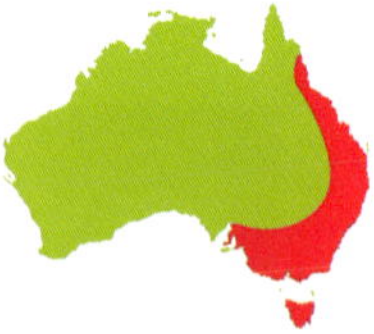

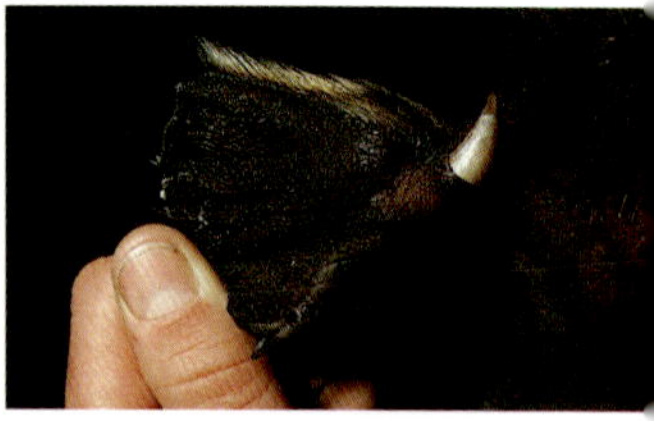

PETER MARSACK/LT

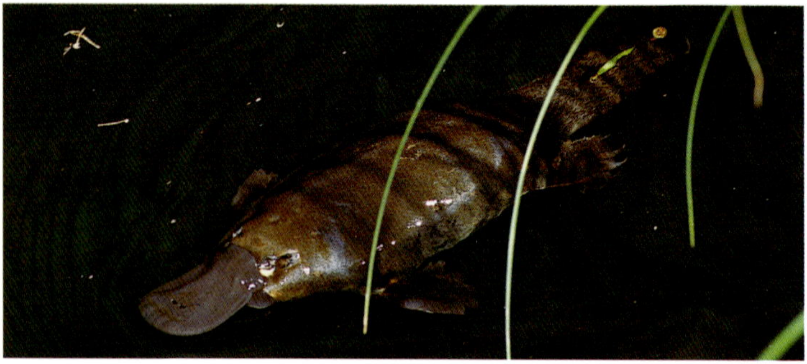

HANS AND JUDY BESTE/LT

Symptoms

A puncture-like wound producing severe pain and swelling for several days.

First Aid

- Restrict movement of affected limb—have victim lie still.
- Use an ice pack or local anaesthetic cream to reduce pain.
- Seek medical aid.

POISONOUS PLANTS ★-★★★

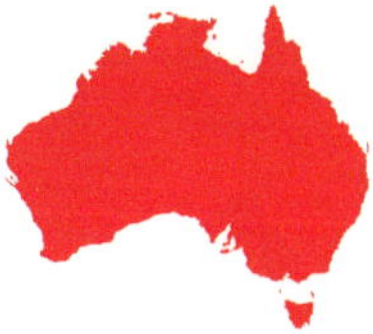

MANY PLANTS commonly found in gardens or in bushland adjacent to suburban areas are poisonous if eaten. It is beyond the scope of this book to include these, especially as there are no common features to distinguish poisonous from non-poisonous plants. Some are regarded as weeds while others are prized as colourful ornamental plants. People with young children should be aware of those plants that may be a danger and remove them from the garden. A few of the more common ones are: Angel's Trumpet, Poinsettia, oleanders and foxgloves. All parts of these plants are poisonous. (*Continued over*)

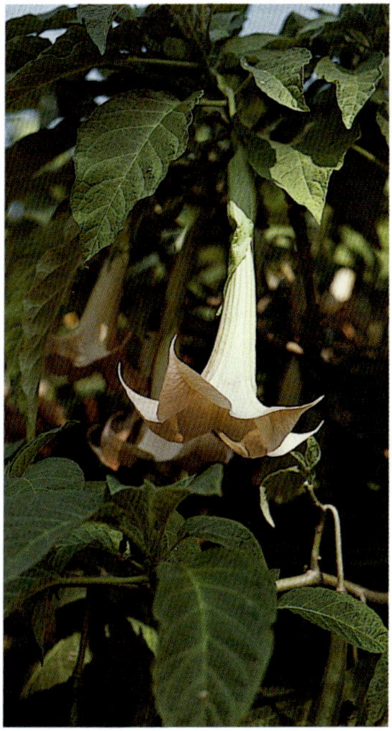

DENISE GREIG

Angel's Trumpet

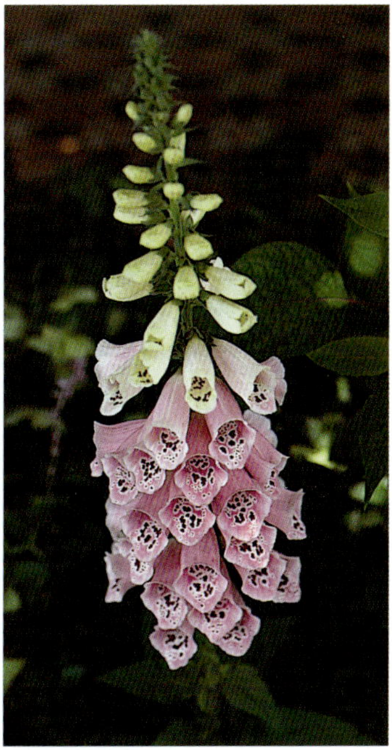

DENISE GREIG

Foxglove

P POISONOUS PLANTS ★★

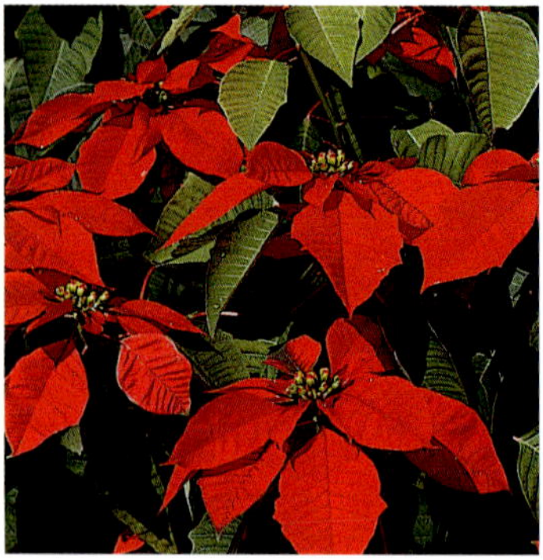

DENISE GREIG

Poinsettia

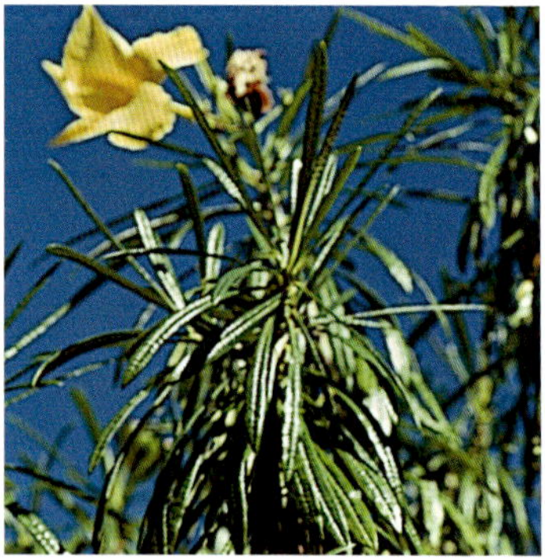

DENISE GREIG

Yellow Oleander

Symptoms

The symptoms are varied and depend upon the type of plant that has been eaten: burning of the mouth, nausea, diarrhoea, delirium, irregular pulse and convulsions are some of the symptoms that may occur.

Crawling or toddling children are most at risk of eating pieces of plants. Fortunately, many poisonous plants are bitter to taste, so children will quickly spit them out before thoroughly chewing or swallowing. With young children the symptoms may only be a crying child, or plant remains in the mouth or near the child.

First Aid

- In case of contact with skin or eyes, wash with clean running water.
- Remove any remaining plant material from the mouth and wash mouth out.
- Contact the Poisons Information Centre (page 7) for advice.
- Seek immediate medical aid if the victim is unconscious, having breathing difficulties or fitting.

RHUS ★★

(Scarlet Rhus)

Small deciduous tree or shrub 5–8m high. Brilliant scarlet to crimson foliage in autumn. Each leaf comprised of 9–15 small pointed leaflets, each 5–10cm long, drooping slightly. Very small pale yellow flowers. Originated in China and Japan; brought into Australia as an attractive ornamental plant. All parts are dangerous. Do not touch this plant. Do not burn any part of the plant as the smoke carries the toxic oil. Contact your Council regarding removal. Suburbs or adjacent bushland.

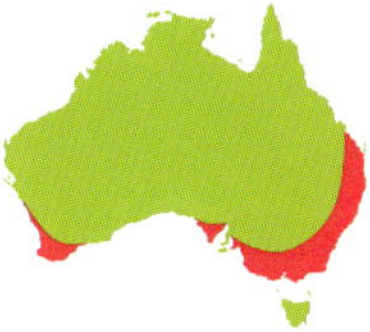

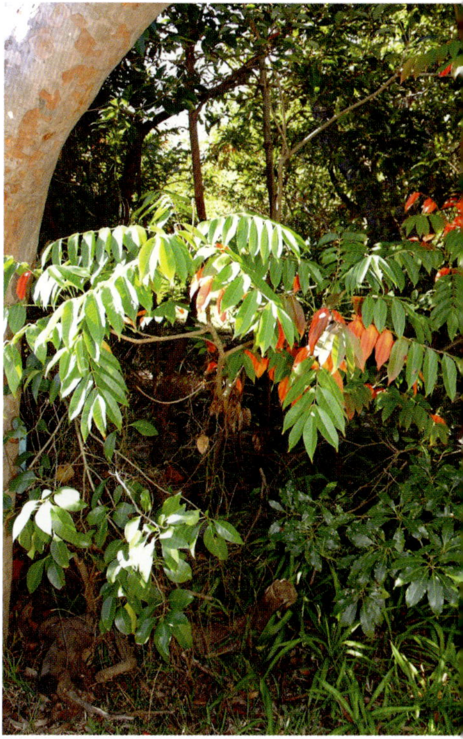

GEOFF SWAN

Symptoms

Severe skin irritation. All parts of this tree are poisonous.

First Aid

- Wash skin with clean running water.
- If eaten, follow first aid for Poisonous Plants (see page 92).

S

SCORPIONS ★★

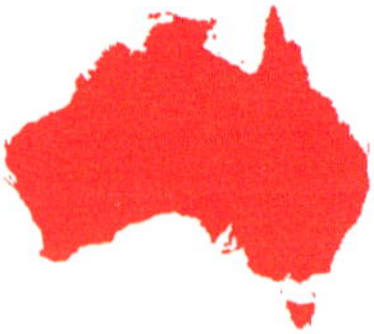

2–12cm long. All scorpions have a pair of claws, eight legs and a sting on the tail that can strike repeatedly over the scorpion's back at a predator or prey. Brown to reddish or black. Eat insects and other arthropods. Most are active at night, hiding in burrows or under stones during the day. Found in warm countries in many parts of the world.

ROB VALENTIC

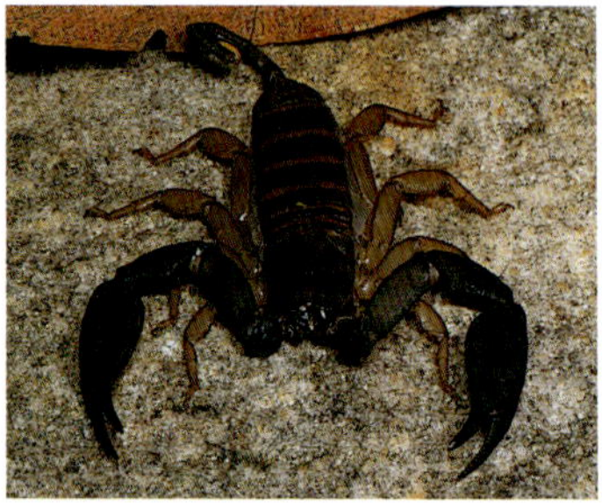

A rock-living scorpion

ROB VALENTIC

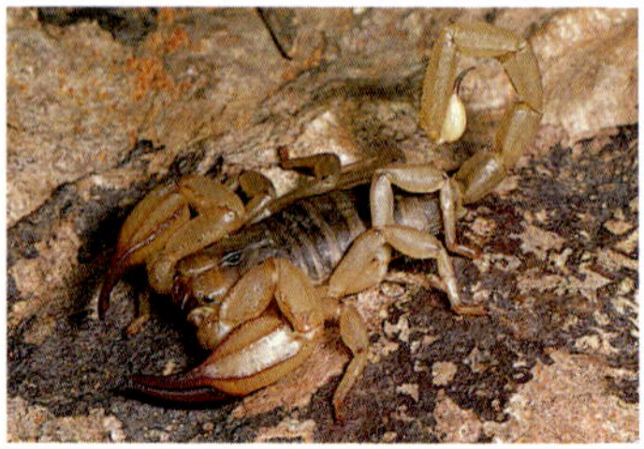

An arid-region scorpion

Symptoms

Local pain and swelling for a few days. Occasionally there may be nausea and headaches.

First Aid

- Apply ice pack/cold compress to reduce swelling.
- Apply local anaesthetic cream.
- Seek medical aid if symptoms persist.

SEA LIZARD ★★★

(Glaucus)

1–3cm long. Slug-like with three 'limbs' on each side of the body, each with numerous finger-like pieces. Floats in surface waters with blue underside uppermost. Back is white. Coastal waters.

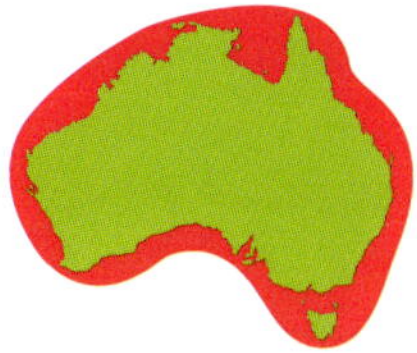

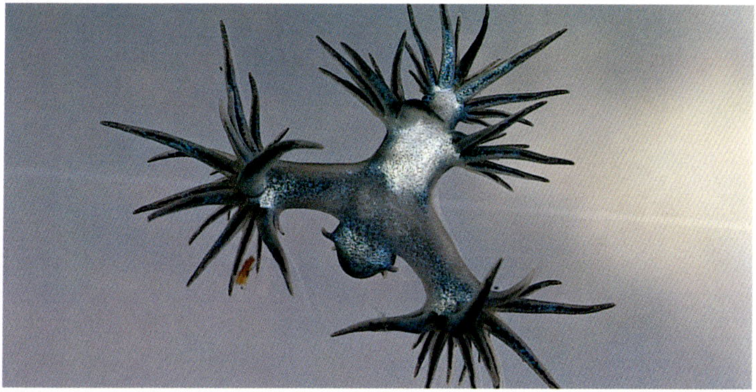

MARK SPENCER

Symptoms

This animal eats microscopic jellyfish, including their venoms. The severity of its stings depends upon what it has eaten recently. Minor irritation or stinging may increase if rubbed and appear as a red blotchy patch. If the stinging is extensive there can be vomiting, diarrhoea, fever and abdominal pains. Usually the pain will increase for 10–15 minutes then subside.

First Aid

- Remove the victim from the water and reassure.
- Apply ice pack or local anaesthetic cream.
- Seek medical aid if symptoms persist or increase.

S SEA SNAKES ★★★★

SEA SNAKES are totally aquatic. They have vertically flattened, often paddle-shaped tails, and valved nostrils situated on top of the head. The majority are dangerously venomous but have small fangs and are reluctant to bite. Three of the more common species are described below.

Symptoms

Usually the bite will be felt and it takes the form of a series of small punctures or lacerations. If envenomation has occurred the symptoms may include muscular pain and weakness, drooping eyelids, blurred vision, difficulty in breathing and swallowing. Death can result from respiratory paralysis.

First Aid

- Remove the victim from the water and keep still and calm.
- Wrap a broad bandage around the bite site and limb using the pressure-immobilisation technique (see page 15).
- Immobilise the bitten limb with a splint.
- Bring transport to the victim if possible.
- Get medical aid as soon as possible.
- Maintain a watch on the victim. If breathing or heart stops begin EAR or CPR (see pages 11–12).

ELEGANT SEA SNAKE

1–2m long. Slender neck and forebody. Pale brown with a dark head and numerous dark bands that are narrow or broken on the sides. In deeper waters between reefs.

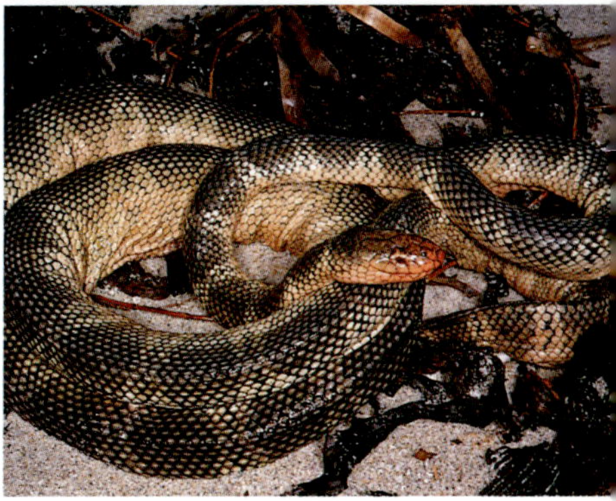

BRAD MARYAN

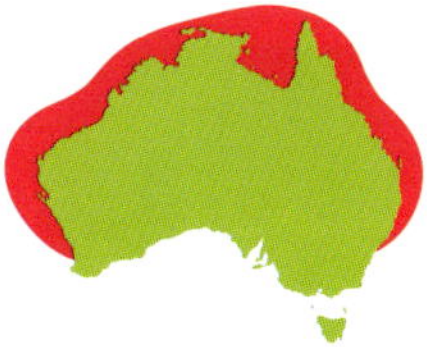

OLIVE SEA SNAKE

1.5–2.2m long. Large and robust. Blackish brown to golden brown, with or without numerous creamy spots, or, in the lighter coloured individuals, scattered dark scales. Common and widespread on reefs of northern Australia. Extends down to the central coasts of NSW and WA.

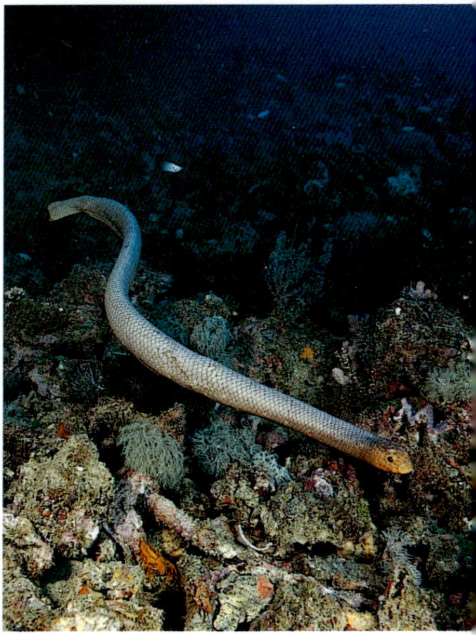

BECCA SAUNDERS

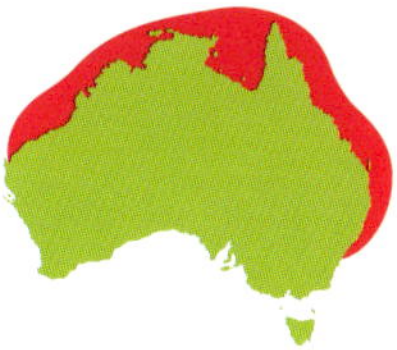

S SEA SNAKES ★★★★

YELLOW-BELLIED SEA SNAKE

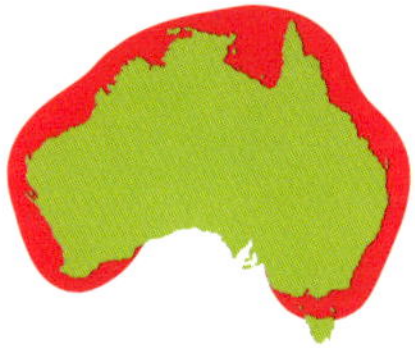

0.5–1m long. Upper half of the body black, lower half pale brown or yellow, with the two colours sharply separated. Tail yellow to cream with black spots. An oceanic snake that occurs almost all round the coast, and is often washed ashore by storms.

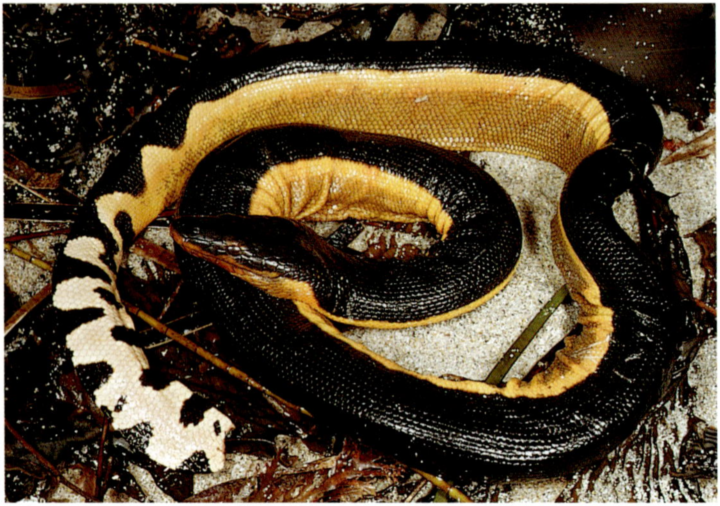

BRAD MARYAN

First Aid — see page 96

SEA URCHINS ★★★

(Sea Eggs)

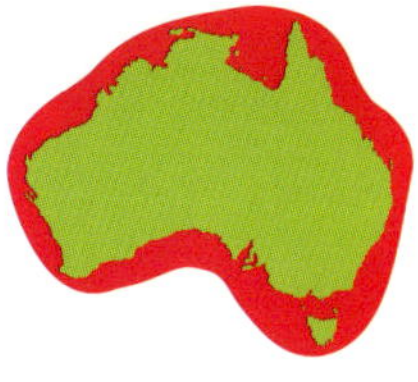

1–20cm in diameter. Various colours, shapes and sizes. Mostly globe shaped. Covered in short or long needle-like, brittle spines. Also have short, flower-like snapping organs that sting. Coastal areas among seaweed or under ledges in rock pools. (*Continued over*)

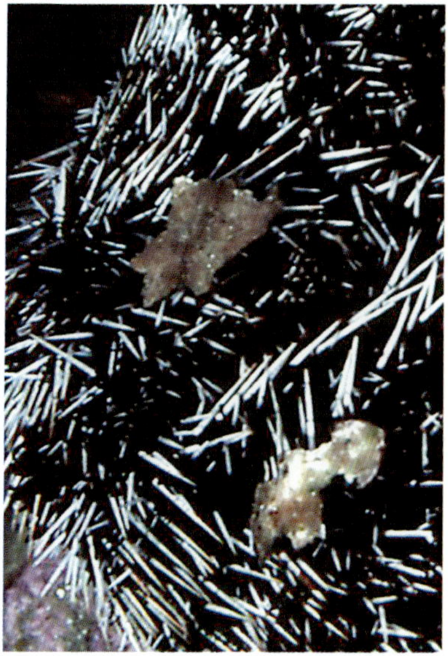

SANDY JACKA

Black Sea Urchin

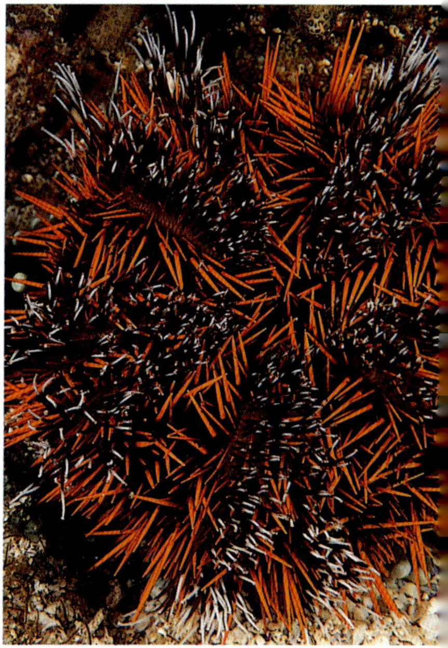

BECCA SAUNDERS

Flower Urchin

S SEA URCHINS

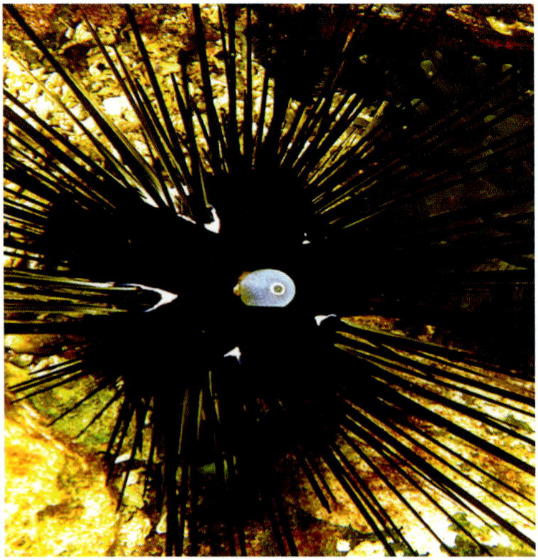

NEIL VINCENT

Needle-shaped Sea Urchin

Symptoms

Handling or treading on sea urchins can cause spines to break off and penetrate flesh, causing immediate severe pain lasting from one to four hours. Swelling and inflammation may become numb around wound and there may be a black discolouration of the punctures.

First Aid

- Immerse wound in hot water to reduce pain.
- Removal of spines from flesh must be done vertically, with no sideways movement, as they are very brittle and break off easily.
- Encourage the victim to move the affected limb—activity appears to ease the pain.
- Seek medical aid.

SHARKS ★★★★

THERE ARE more than 165 species of shark in Australian waters. Do not torment, provoke or handle them. Attacks are known to occur at dusk or in murky, cloudy water. Sharks known to have been involved in attacks on people are the Great White Shark, the Tiger Shark, the Bull Shark and the Oceanic White-tipped Shark.

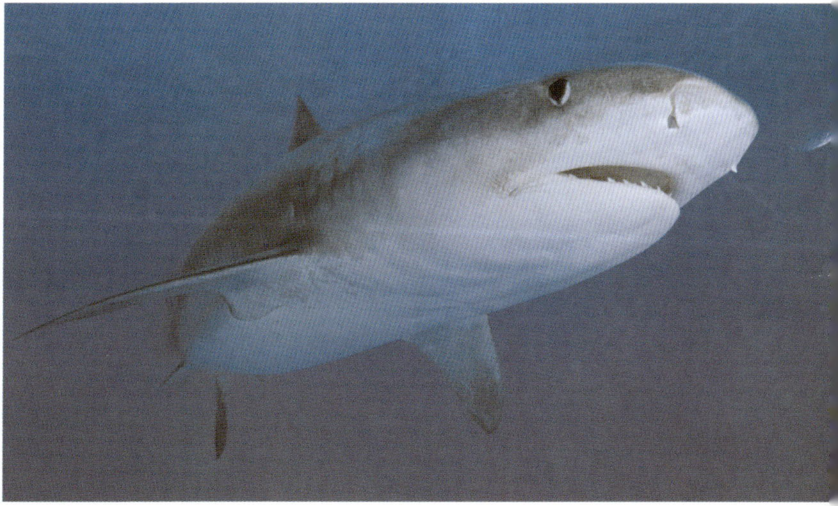

MARINETHEMES.COM/KELVIN AITKEN

Tiger Shark

Symptoms

Lacerated limbs and body, severed limbs, major bleeding, death.

First Aid

- Your priority must be to stop the bleeding (see page 14).
- Treat victim for shock (see page 16).
- Bring medical aid to the victim as quickly as possible.

S SHARKS ★★★★

GREAT WHITE SHARK

(White Pointer, White Death, Great White)

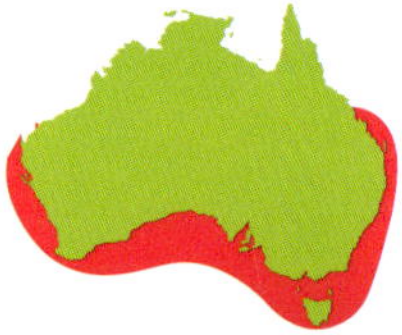

Up to 6m long. Torpedo-shaped body, pointed snout. Large pectoral and first dorsal fins, crescent-shaped tail. Black eyes. Light to dark grey above, paler on the sides. Belly white. Fast-moving shark that is more of a biter than an eater. People are usually tasted and spat out. Presumably mistaken for seals.

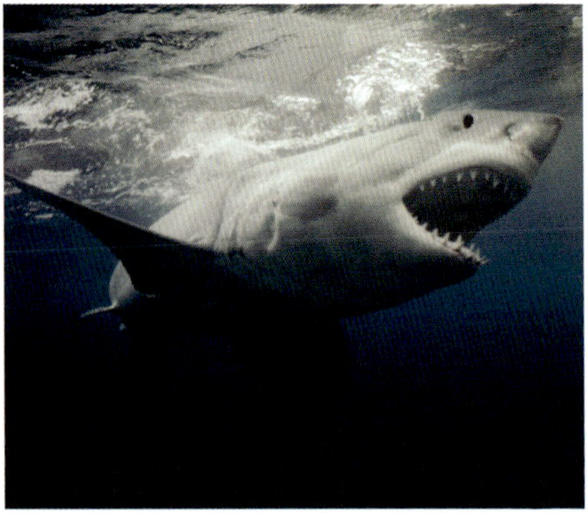

MARINETHEMES.COM/KELVIN AITKEN

TIGER SHARK

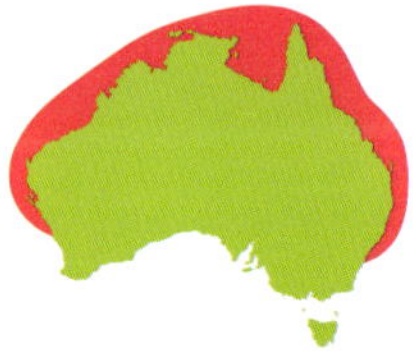

Up to 5m long. Broad head and blunt snout. Dark eyes. Grey, with prominent blotching in juveniles that becomes vertical banding in adults, fading with age. A scavenger in shallow waters, it will eat almost anything it comes across.

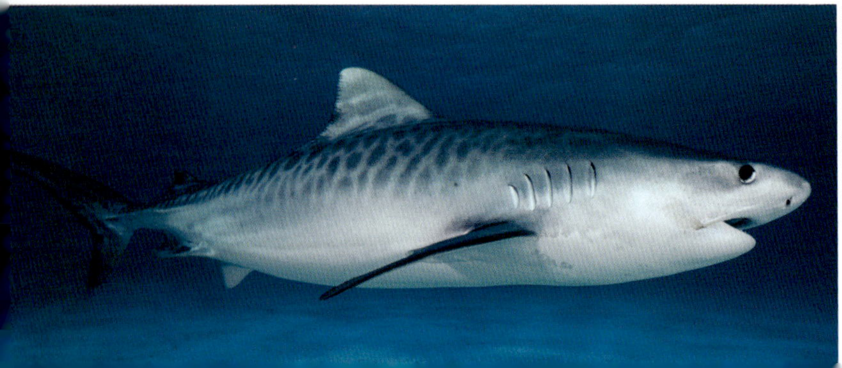

MARINETHEMES.COM/KELVIN AITKEN

OCEANIC WHITE-TIP

(Oceanic White-tipped Shark)

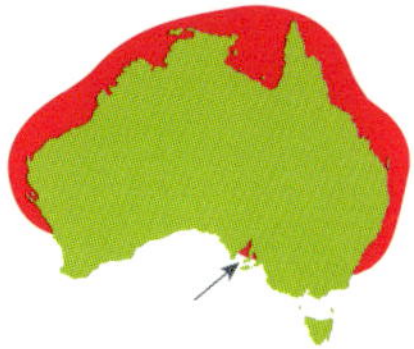

Up to 3.5m long. Olive brown to bronze, paler below, with long paddle-shaped pectoral fins and a long first dorsal fin. Blotchy white colouration on tip of pectoral and first dorsal fins. Second dorsal fin has a black tip. Offshore in open waters. Ocean-going shark that swimmers rarely encounter. However, very inquisitive and may circle swimmers or divers.

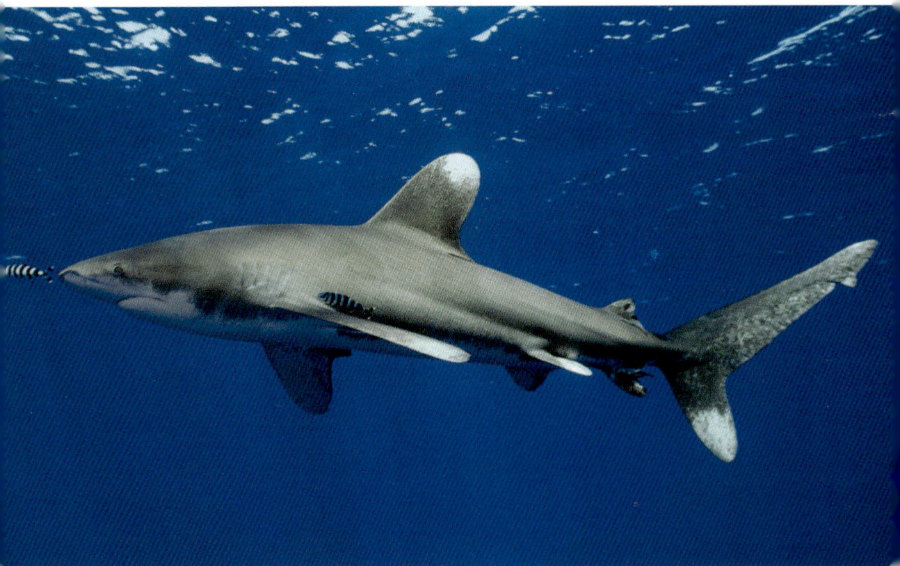

MARINETHEMES.COM/KELVIN AITKEN

First Aid — see page 101

SHARKS ★★★★

BULL SHARK

(Cub Shark, Zambesi, Ground Shark)

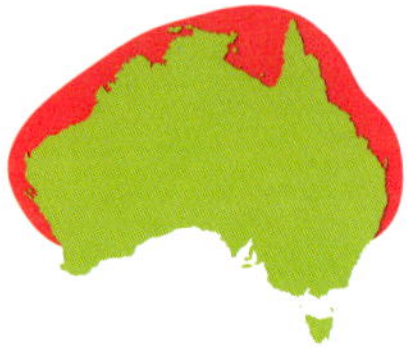

Up to 3.5m long. Stout body, short, blunt snout with a small eye. Grey above and pale below. Aggressive. Northern Australia, as far south as Swan River, WA, and Clarence River, NSW. Inhabits rivers, lakes, estuaries and shallow water. Avoid swimming in murky water near river mouths or in estuaries.

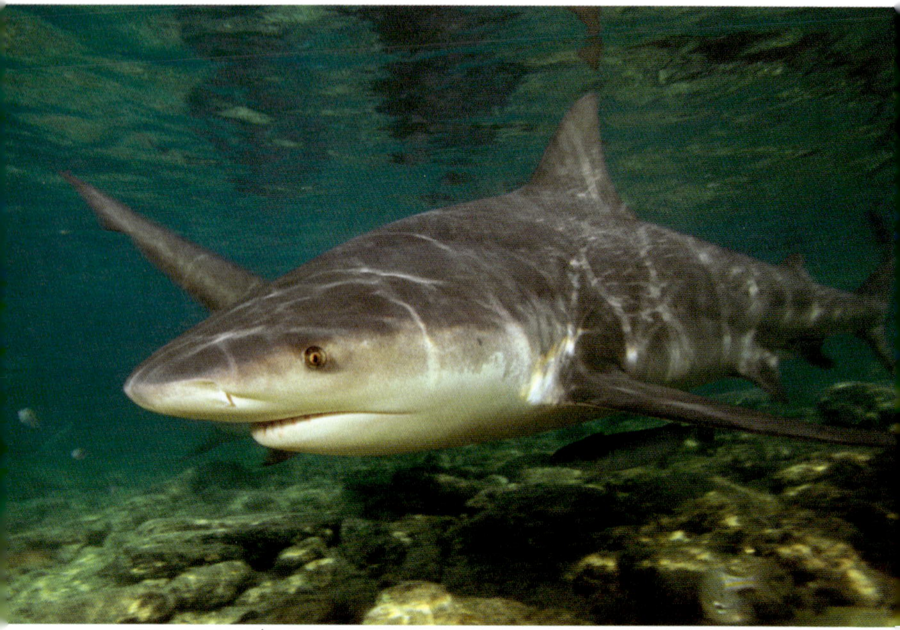

MARINETHEMES.COM/MARK CONLIN

First Aid — see page 101

THE MAJORITY of shells are formed by living animals called molluscs, and provide shelter for the soft-bodied inhabitant, some of which are very dangerous. The shells are made of calcium carbonate and the mollusc inside will add material to the shell so that it grows as the animal does.

CONE SHELLS ★★★★

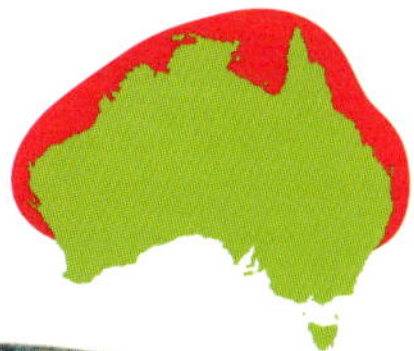

2–12cm long. Conical in shape, with many patterns and colours. Shell often covered with a thin horny layer that blurs or hides the patterns and colours. All cone shells are predatory and use a barbed dart to kill prey. Only a few are regarded as dangerous to people, but 25% of persons stung by these have died as a result. There is no safe way to hold live cone shells. The barbed sting can penetrate light clothing. Coastal areas.

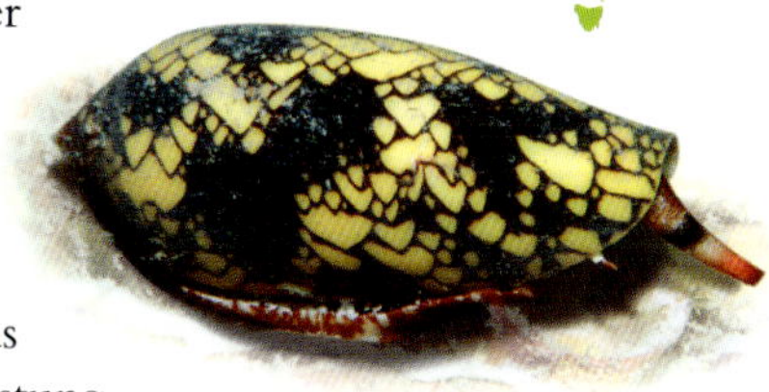

MARINETHEMES.COM/CLAY BRYCE

Court Cone

Symptoms

Sting may or may not be painful. Numbness of extremities, tingling around lips and mouth, blurring of vision, paralysis, coma and death.

First Aid

- Check breathing and pulse and if necessary commence EAR or CPR immediately (see pages 11–12).
- Apply a pressure bandage and immobilise the limb (see page 16).
- Seek medical aid.

RAZOR CLAM ★

(Razor Shell)

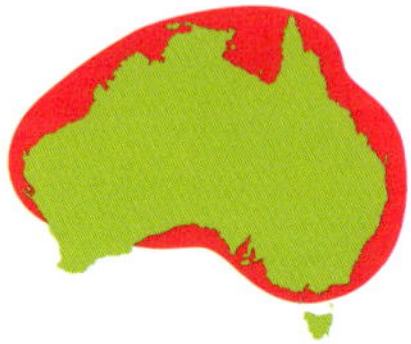

40–50cm long. Two wedge-shaped, joined shells. Purple–brown to dark brown. Coastal areas except for Tas and southern WA. Buries itself in mud or sand with the thin, sharp, wide end uppermost, often protruding.

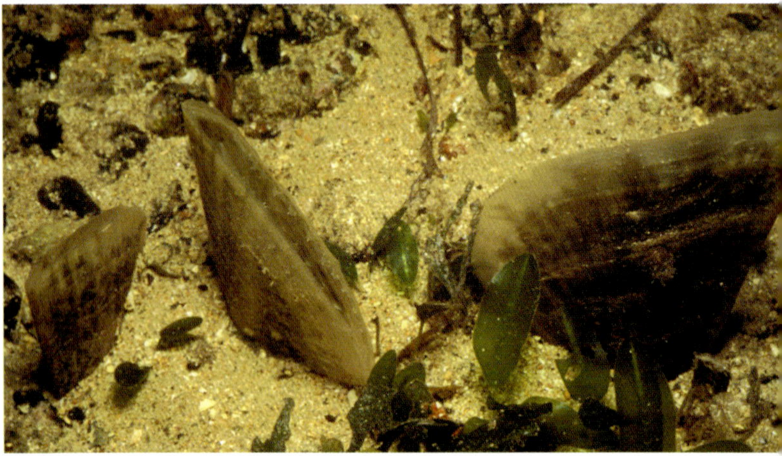

KAREN GOWLETT-HOLMES

A cluster of razor clams protruding from sand.

Symptoms

Gash, usually on the foot, caused by treading on protruding shell. Sharp pain, usually accompanied by profuse bleeding.

First Aid

- Wash wound and control bleeding (see page 14).
- Apply a dressing.

SHRIMP, MANTIS ★

(Split Thumbs)

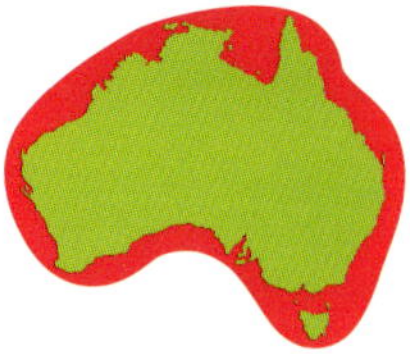

1–40cm long. Prawn-like, with strong claws like those of a praying mantis, and six pairs of legs. One species has club-like claws that are used to crush prey. Others have spear-like claws that impale prey. Aggressive predators that dart out from their burrows and crush or spear victims with their strong claws. Coastal waters. More common in tropical areas. Live in burrows in sand flats and coral.

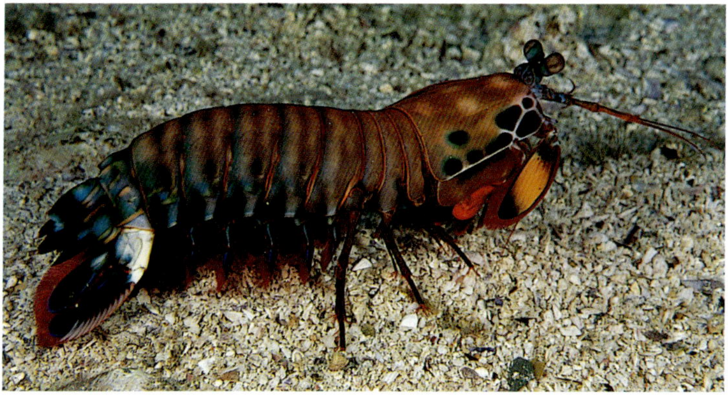

BECCA SAUNDERS

Symptoms

A bruised and blackened or badly slashed thumb or finger.

First Aid

- If a laceration, wash and apply antiseptic cream and a dressing.
- If bruised or crushed, apply an ice pack/cold compress.

SNAKES

WITH OVER 150 described species of snake in Australia it is inevitable that most people will meet one at some stage. Fortunately, the majority are not dangerous. However, identification of different species can be tricky, involving colour pattern, distribution and certain scale characteristics. As using the scale characteristics involves close examination of the animal, we have not included these in this book.

Colour helps identify some species, but is notoriously unreliable for others. For example, the Common Brown Snake can be light tan to black in colour, with or without speckles or bands. People with little or no experience in handling snakes should leave all snakes alone. Snakes bite people only when they feel threatened due to being handled, provoked, molested or otherwise interfered with.

Antivenom is available for the treatment of bites by dangerously venomous snakes.

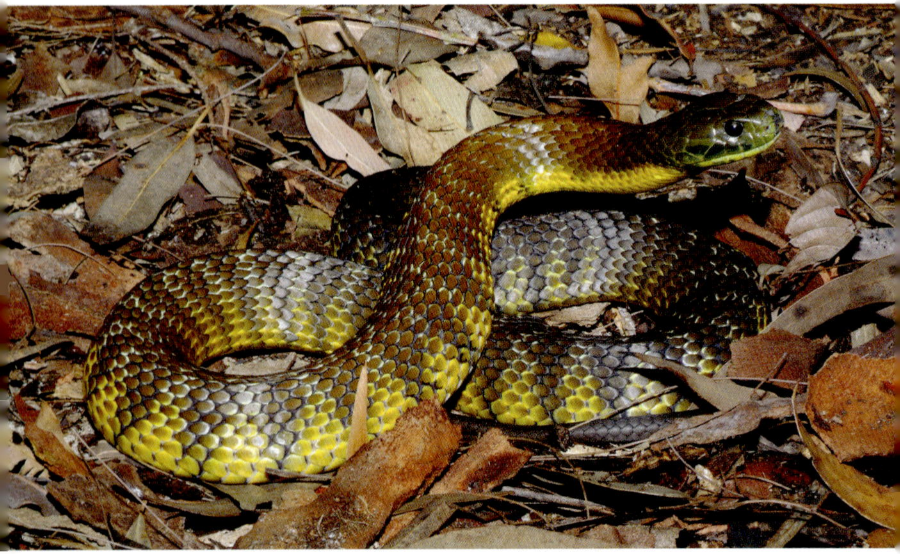

Eastern Tiger Snake GEOFF SWAN

Symptoms

Snake bites are sometimes painless and may not be noticed. Most bites involving serious envenomation cause some or all of the following symptoms: severe headache, nausea and vomiting, abdominal pain, drooping eyelids, difficulty breathing, blurred vision, desire to urinate or defecate, paralysis, unconsciousness and death.

First Aid

Do

- Keep the victim still and calm.
- Immediately apply a pressure-immobilisation bandage to the bite site and wrap it around as much of the limb as possible (see page 15).
- Immobilise the bitten limb with a splint.
- Bring transport to the victim if possible.
- Get medical aid to the victim as soon as possible.
- Maintain a watch on the victim. If breathing or heart stops, commence EAR or CPR (see pages 11–12).

Do not

- Try to catch or kill the snake.
- Cut or suck the bite.
- Wash the bite.
- Place Condy's Crystals on the bite.
- Use tourniquets.
- Let the victim drink stimulants such as coffee or alcohol.

BROWN SNAKES ★★★★

BROWN SNAKES are responsible for most snake bites in Australia (they also cause the most deaths). Of the seven recognised species in Australia, six are dangerously venomous. Between them they cover almost all of Australia except Tas.

It is not possible to identify these snakes with certainty without some knowledge of the animals. They are all fast moving and active during the day, but also move about at night during hot weather. They range from 60cm to 2.2m long, with narrow heads and moderately large eyes.

In colour they range from light tan, through every shade of brown to almost black. Some have orange or yellow colouration. They may be banded, speckled, or have a darker herringbone pattern or scattered black scales, and some have a glossy black head. The belly is white to pale yellow with orange blotches.

Generally shy, they become aggressive if provoked or threatened, raising the head and forebody and striking repeatedly.

Symptoms (First Aid — see page 109)

Bite can be hard to see and there is little or no pain. Victim may develop severe headaches, nausea and vomiting, blood-clotting defects and paralysis. Death can follow.

EASTERN OR COMMON BROWN SNAKE

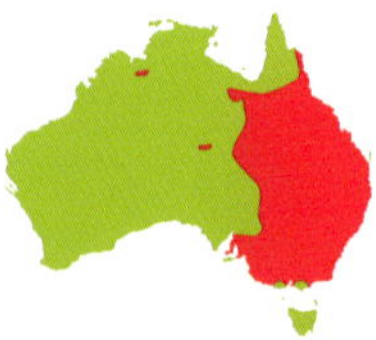

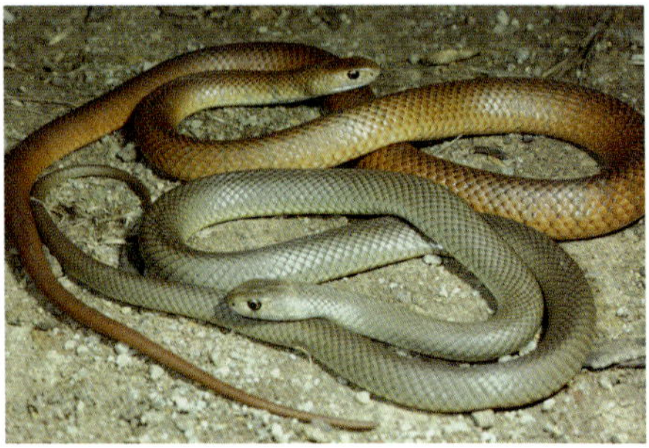

JOHN WOMBEY

INGRAM'S BROWN SNAKE

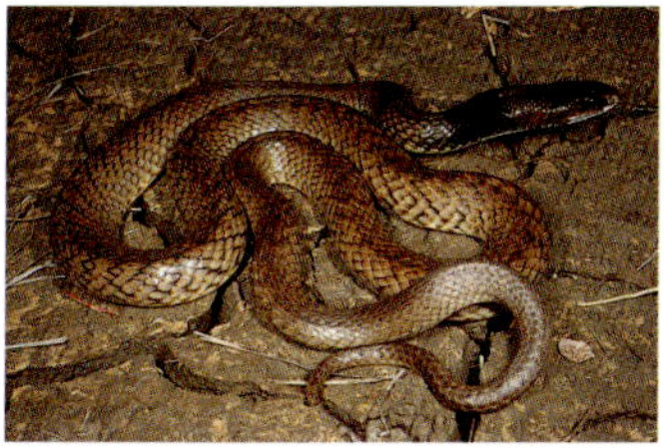

BRAD MARYAN

DUGITE

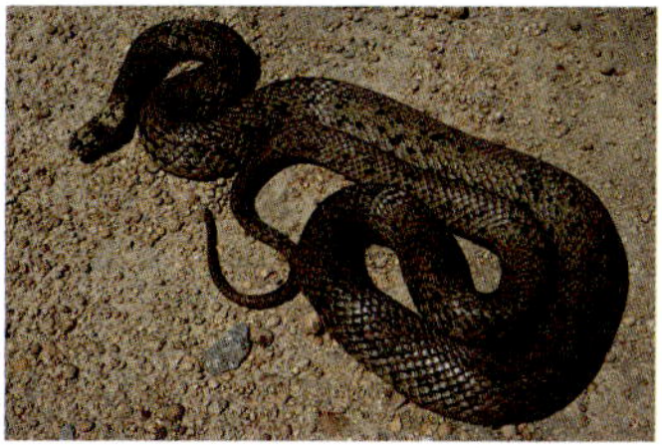

BRAD MARYAN

PENINSULA BROWN SNAKE

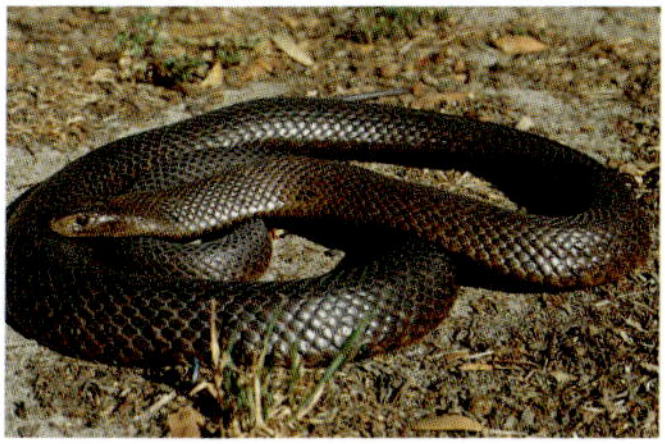

BRIAN BUSH

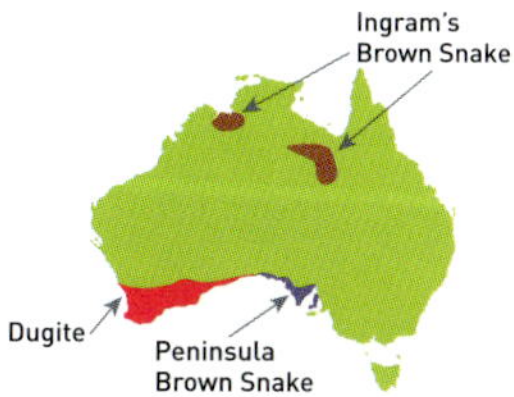

WESTERN BROWN SNAKE OR GWARDAR

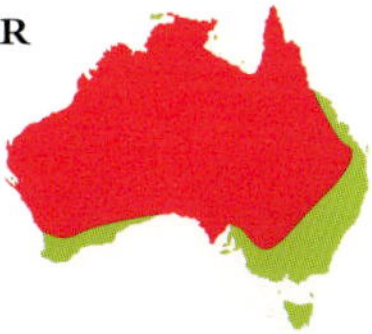

ROB VALENTIC

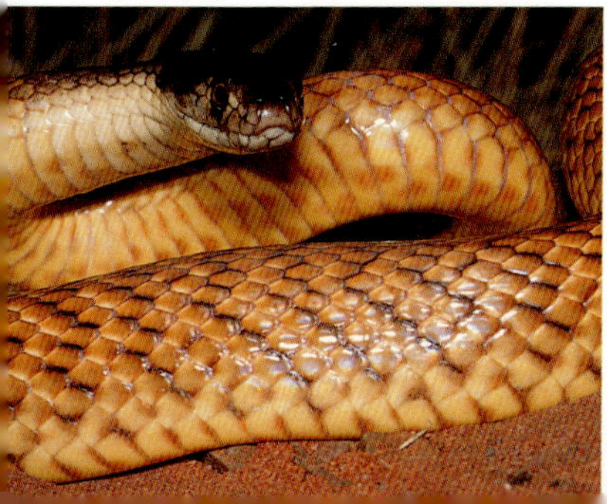

SPECKLED BROWN SNAKE

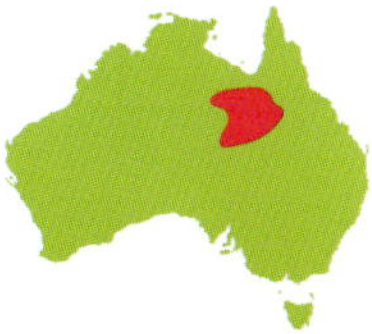

ROB VALENTIC

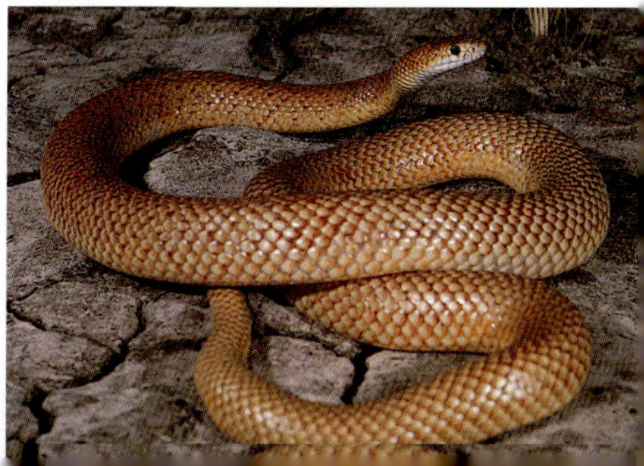

DEATH ADDERS ★★★★

FOUR RECOGNISED species occur through much of Australia. All are short (0.5–1m long), robust snakes with a broad head which is distinct from the neck, and a short, thin tail which ends in a soft spine. These snakes have large fangs. They are infrequently encountered and rely on camouflage and not moving to avoid detection.

Symptoms (First Aid — see page 109)
Local pain and swelling, headaches, drooping eyelids, breathing difficulties, paralysis and muscle damage. Death can follow.

DESERT DEATH ADDER
Light reddish brown to red, with numerous narrow yellowish bands.

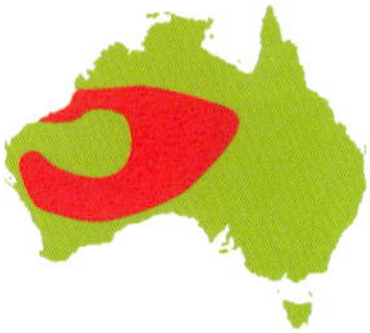

ROB VALENTIC

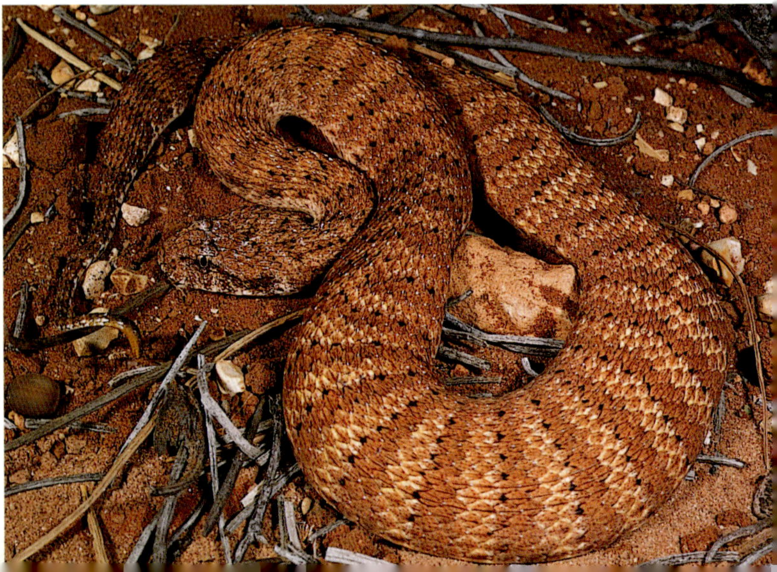

COMMON DEATH ADDER

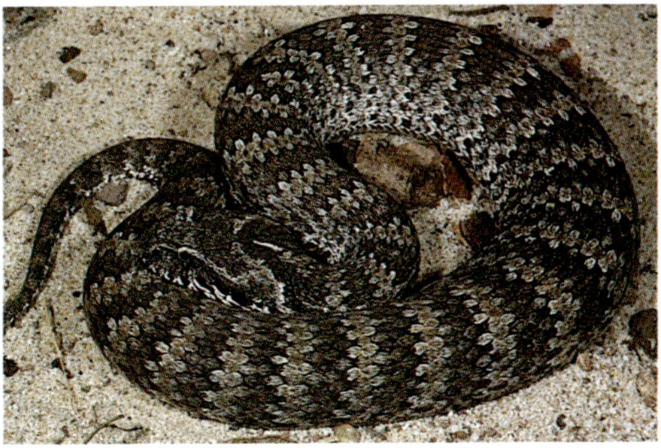

GEOFF SWAN

NORTHERN DEATH ADDER

Grey, red–brown to dark brown with pale cross bands that are dark edged. Also on Torres Strait islands.

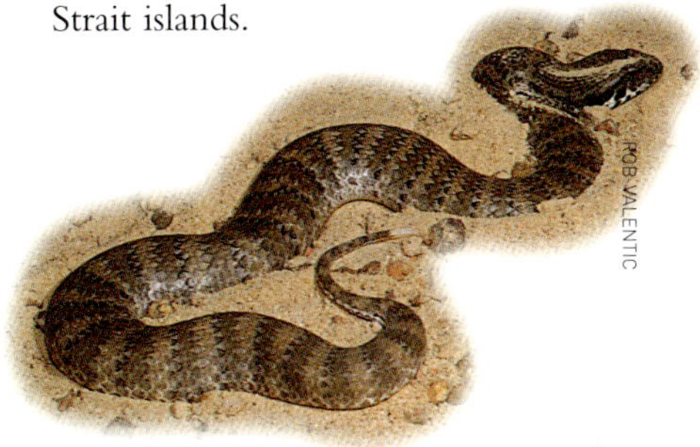

ROB VALENTIC

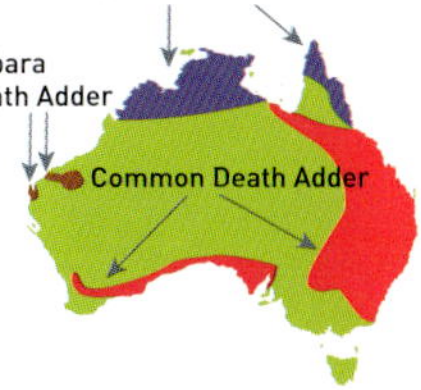

PILBARA DEATH ADDER

Reddish brown with either dark or pale cross bands. Some individuals have a black head.

ROB VALENTIC

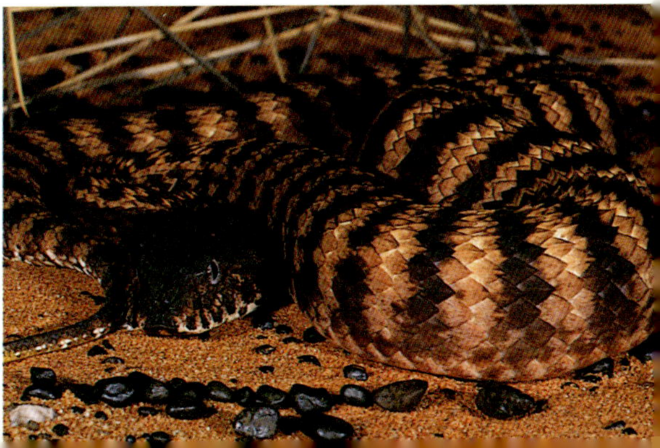

TIGER SNAKES ★★★★

(Eastern Tiger Snake, Black Tiger Snake, Western Tiger Snake)

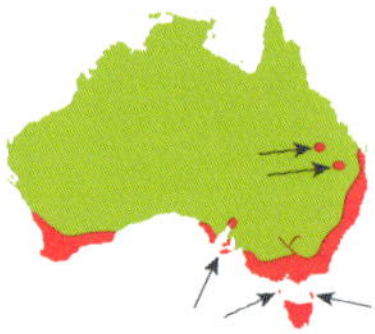

90cm–2m long. Robust snake with a broad head. Colour varies from black, grey and brown to yellow, with or without distinct yellowish bands. In some areas (notably SA and Bass Strait islands) Tiger Snakes are usually entirely black. Eastern and southern coasts including Tas and the Bass Strait islands. Also found in SA in the Flinders Ranges, and Eyre and Yorke peninsulas and offshore islands, and south-western WA. Not aggressive unless provoked. Will flatten neck before striking and tend to strike low to the ground.

Symptoms (First Aid — see page 109)

Painful bite, often with redness and swelling. Headaches, nausea and vomiting, and abdominal pain usually follow, as will paralysis, muscle damage, bleeding and kidney failure. Death can follow.

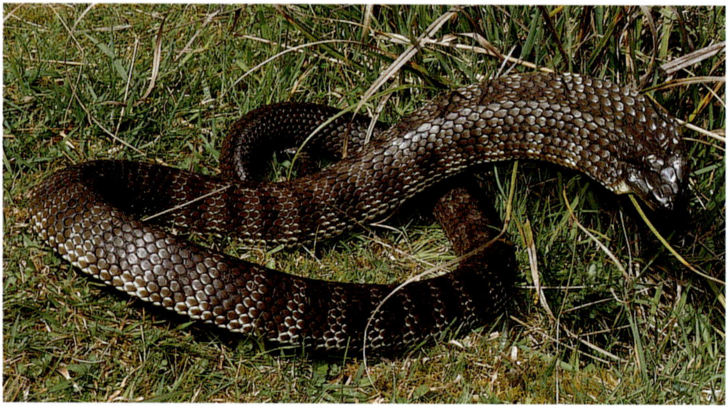

ROB VALENTIC

Eastern Tiger Snake

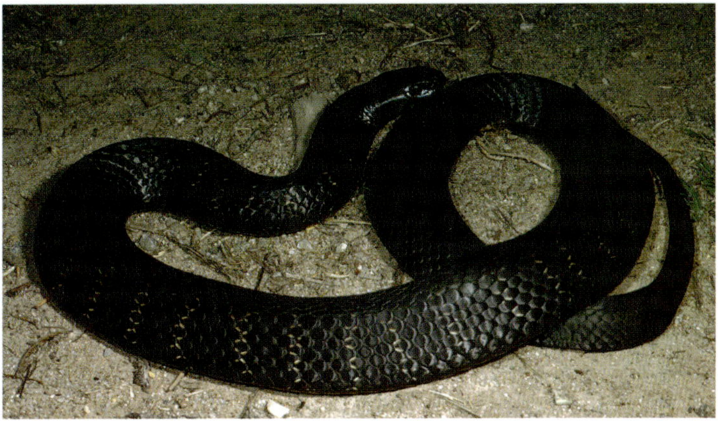
JOHN WOMBEY

Black Tiger Snake

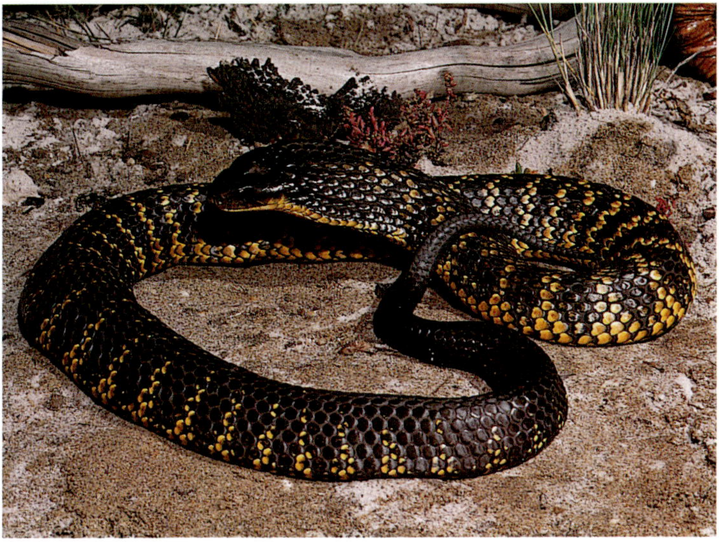
ROB VALENTIC

Western Tiger Snake

COPPERHEAD SNAKES ★★★★

80cm–1.8m long. Solidly built with a small head only slightly distinct from the neck. Found in cool, moist areas. Reluctant to bite, they will hiss loudly and flatten the neck when provoked. There are three species.

Symptoms (First Aid — see page 109)
Local pain and swelling, headaches, drooping eyelids, breathing difficulties, paralysis and muscle damage. Death can follow.

LOWLANDS COPPERHEAD
Brown to almost black with pale yellow or pink lower sides. The lips are only weakly barred.

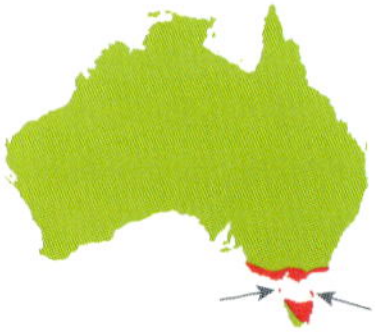

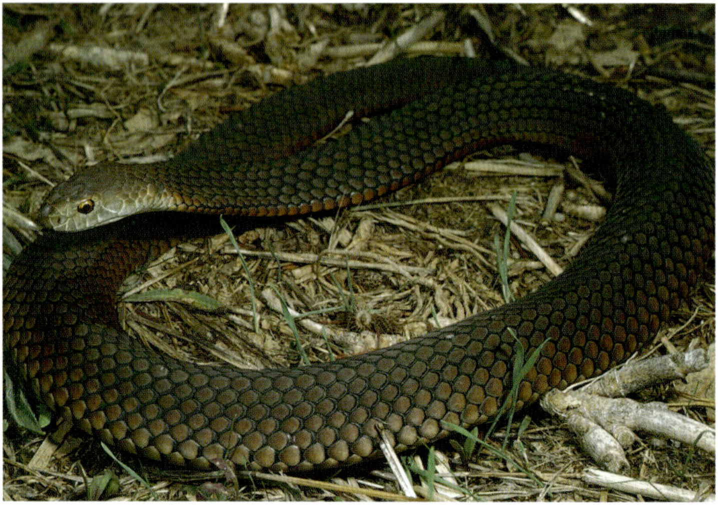

JOHN WOMBEY

HIGHLANDS COPPERHEAD

Dark reddish brown to dark grey with paler or redder lower sides. The lips are prominently barred.

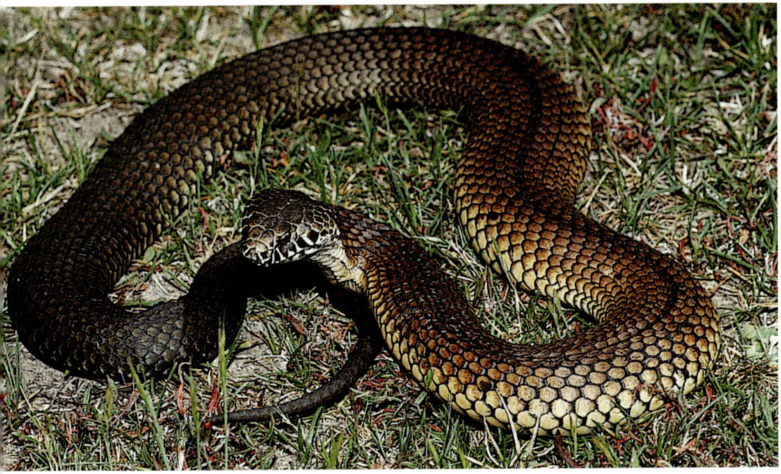

KEN GRIFFITHS

PYGMY COPPERHEAD

Pale brown to dark grey with prominently barred lips.

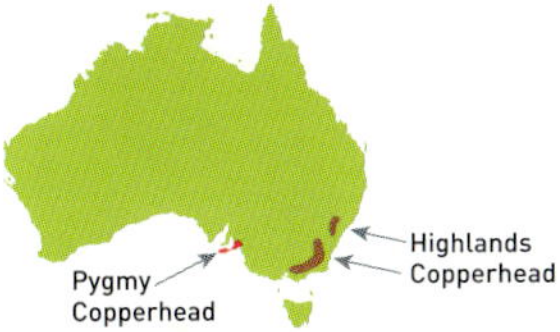

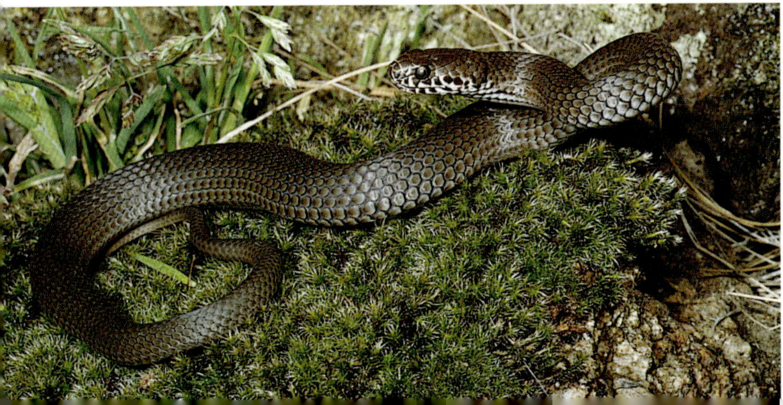

ROB VALENTIC

SNAKES

BLACK SNAKES ★★★★

Five species of black snake are regarded as dangerous. All are large to very large with broad, depressed heads. When threatened they will flatten the neck, presenting the broadest aspect to the aggressor.

Symptoms (First Aid — see page 109)

Painful bite with swelling, muscular weakness and red or brown coloured urine. For Red-bellied Black Snakes there may be headaches, nausea, vomiting, abdominal pain and diarrhoea, but it is not usually regarded as life threatening. The other 'black' snakes can give a painful bite, with muscle damage, kidney failure, bleeding and possible death.

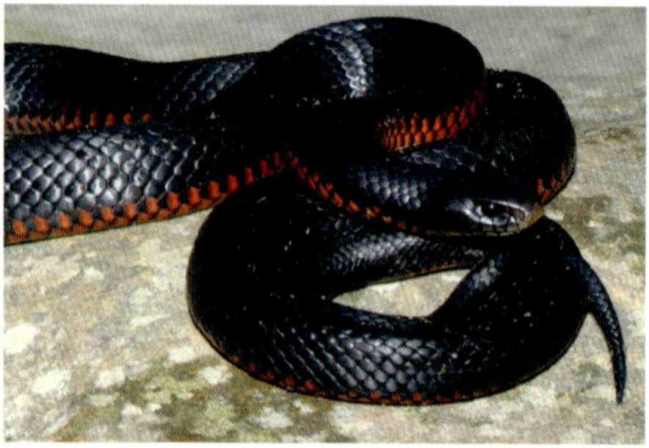

GEOFF SWAN

RED-BELLIED BLACK SNAKE

1–1.8m. Glossy black with red on the lower sides and pink or cream belly. Tip of snout is brown. East coast and adjacent ranges to SA.

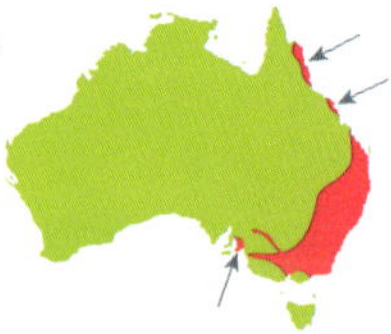

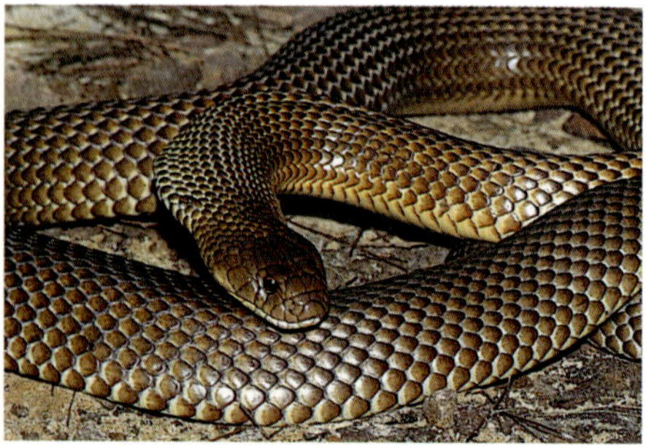

GEOFF SWAN

MULGA (OR KING BROWN) SNAKE

1.5–2.5m. Pale brown to dark brown to reddish brown, often with lighter edges to the scales, giving a reticulated pattern.

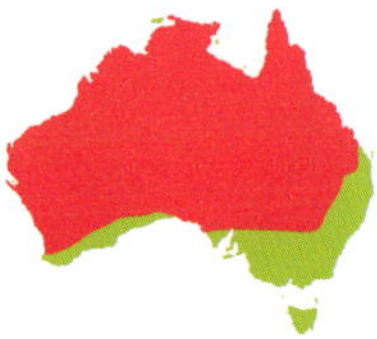

COLLETT'S SNAKE
1–1.5m. Grey or brown to black with irregular cross bands or blotches of pink, red or cream.

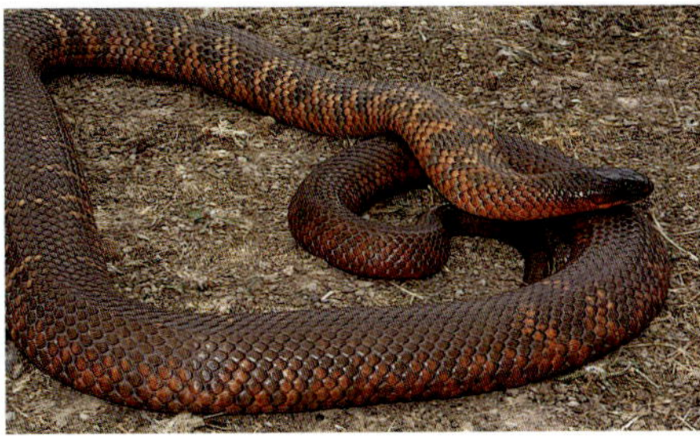
ROB VALENTIC

BUTLER'S (OR SPOTTED) MULGA SNAKE
1–1.6m. Dark grey to black. Most scales have cream centres, giving a patterned appearance.

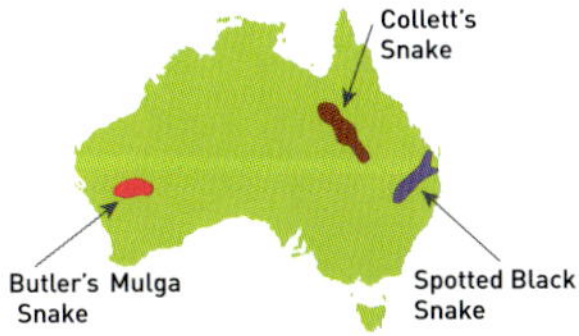

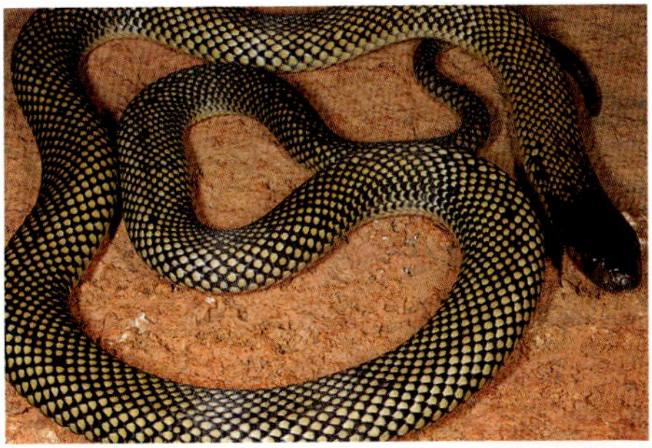
BRAD MARYAN

SPOTTED (OR BLUE-BELLIED) BLACK SNAKE
1–1.5m. Black or brown to grey with or without numerous white spots. Some are white with a black edge to each scale. Belly grey–blue.

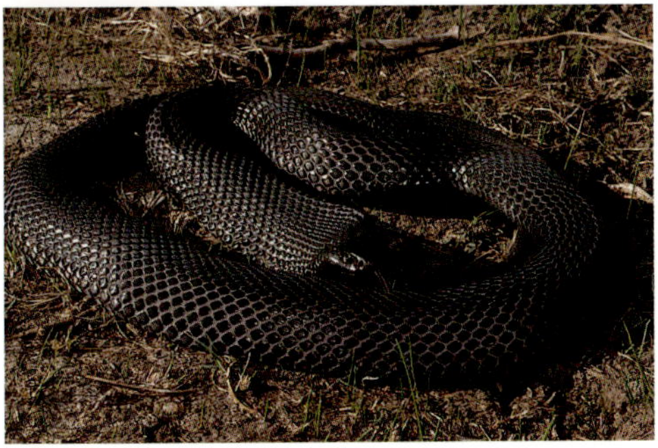
ROB VALENTIC

BROAD-HEADED SNAKES ★★★

Three species of arboreal and rock-climbing snakes that have a broad, flattened head that is distinct from the neck. All can be aggressive if provoked, flattening the head, raising the forebody and striking repeatedly.

Symptoms (First Aid — see page 109)
Local pain and swelling, headache, vomiting, blurred vision, perspiring, difficulty speaking and breathing.

BROAD-HEADED SNAKE
50–90cm. Black with many narrow irregular cross bands of yellow or cream. Sydney region.

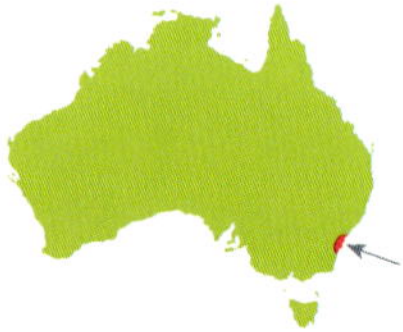

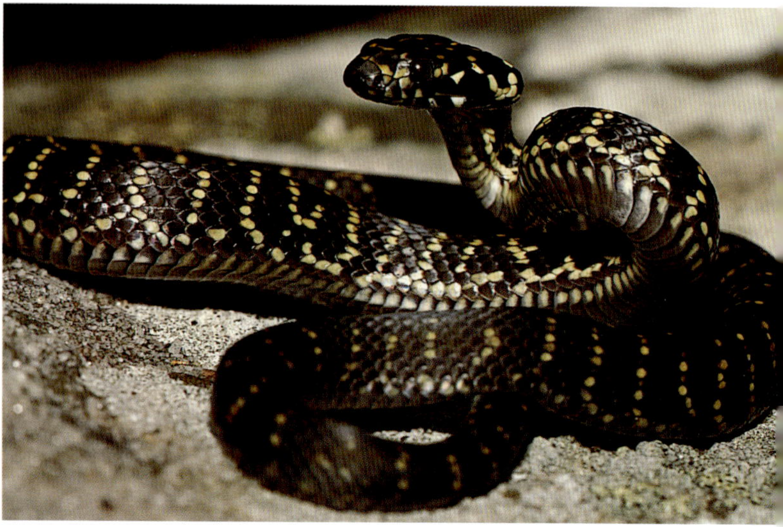

KEN GRIFFITHS

PALE-HEADED SNAKE

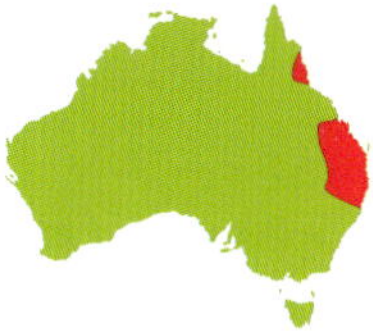

50–80cm. Grey to brownish black with a pale cream band across the neck, edged with a darker band behind. Top of head is grey with blackish flecks.

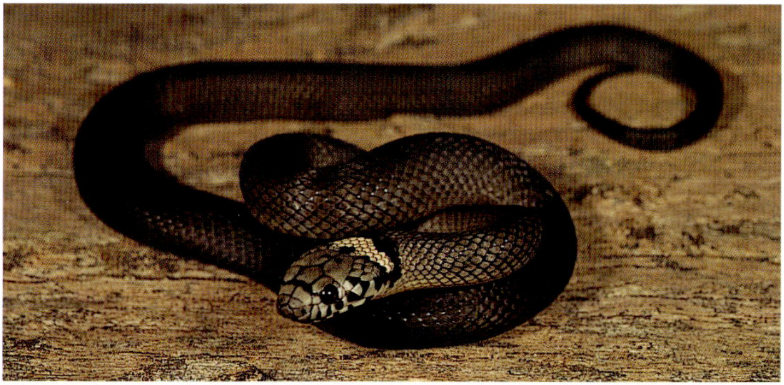

GEOFF SWAN

STEPHEN'S BANDED SNAKE

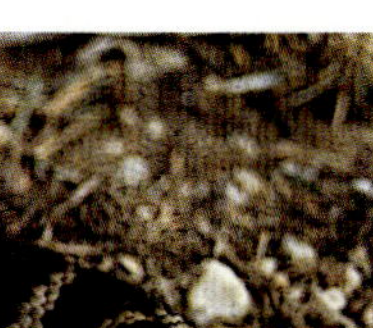

0.8–1.2m. Usually dark grey with many narrow brown or cream bands (occasional unbanded individuals occur). Blotches or bars of black and white on side of head.

GEOFF SWAN

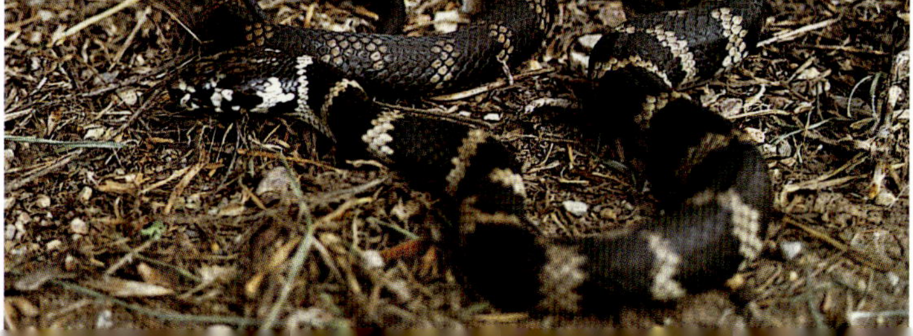

TAIPANS ★★★★

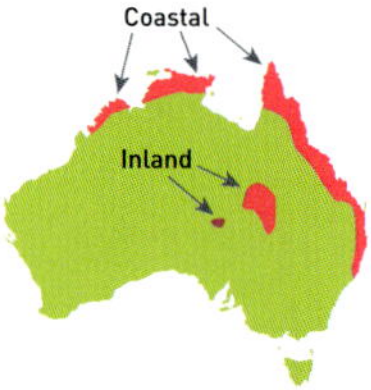

Two very large species with long, narrow heads and large eyes. These snakes have an undeserved reputation for aggressiveness. In reality both avoid confrontations with people, but the Coastal Taipan in particular will defend itself vigorously.

Symptoms (First Aid — see page 109)
There may or may not be pain and swelling at the bite site. Headaches, nausea, vomiting, collapse and paralysis may be rapid developments. Without treatment, death is probable.

INLAND TAIPAN (FIERCE SNAKE, WESTERN TAIPAN, SMALL-SCALED SNAKE)

1–2.5m. Pale yellowish brown to dark brown, usually with dark-edged scales forming a herringbone pattern. Head and neck are glossy black in winter, but this fades in summer. Belly creamy yellow with orange blotches.

ROB VALENTIC

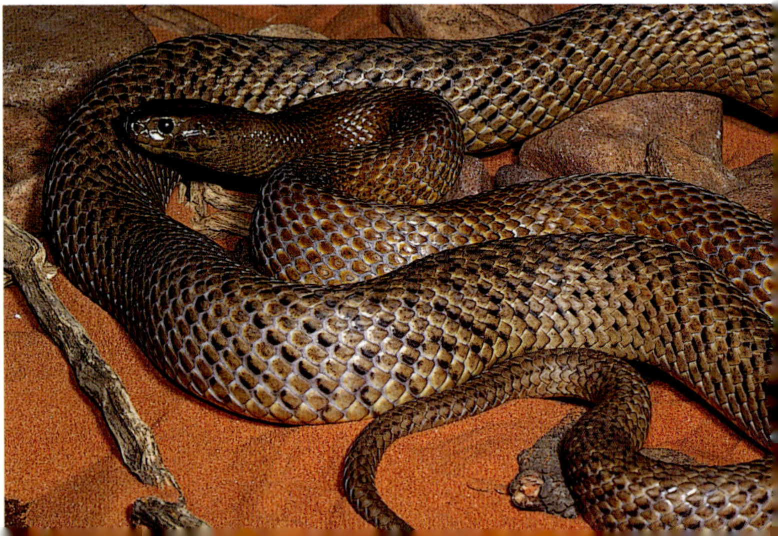

COASTAL TAIPAN

1.5–3m. Yellow–brown to almost black with a pale head and a prominent brow over the eye. Belly cream with yellow or orange blotches.

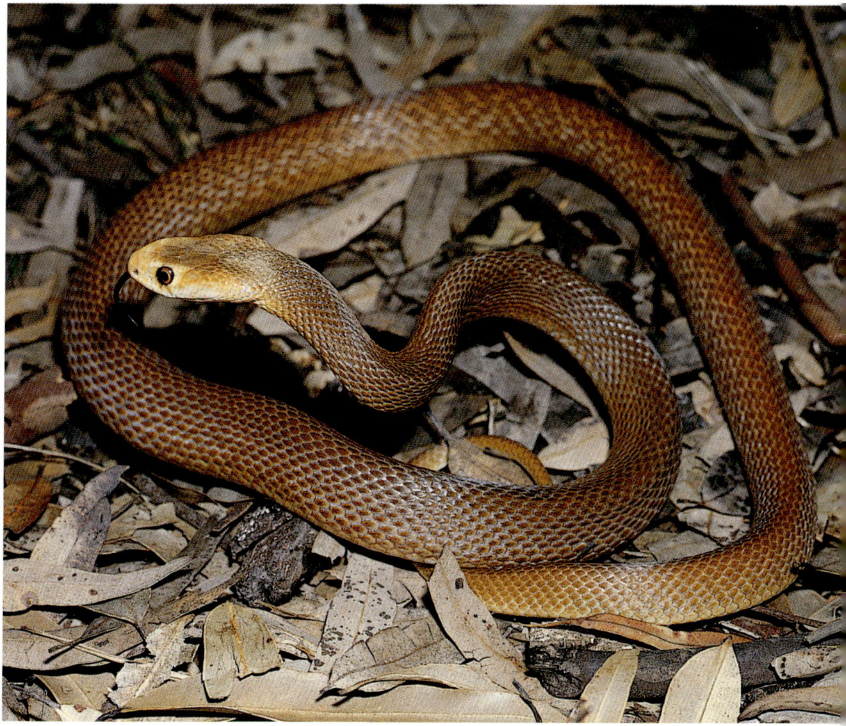

KEN GRIFFITHS

ROUGH-SCALED SNAKE ★★★★

(Clarence River Snake)

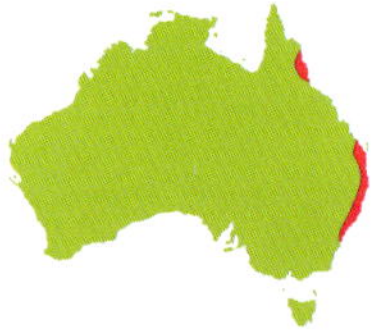

0.7–1m long. Rough, dull scales. Broad head distinct from neck. Large eyes. Yellowish brown to dark brown with dark blotches forming cross bands.

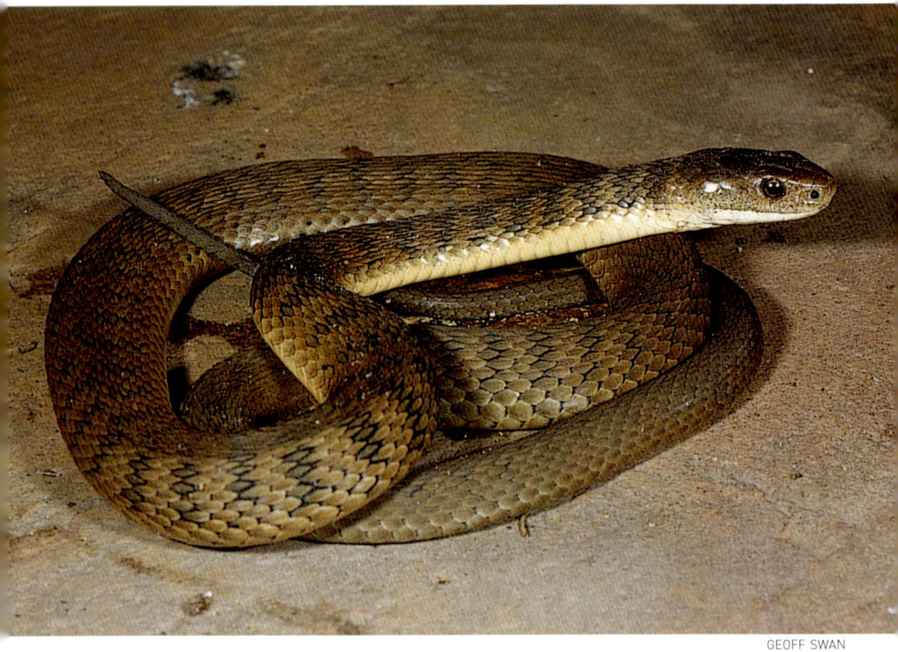

GEOFF SWAN

Symptoms (First Aid — see page 109)

Local pain, swelling, vomiting, blurred vision, diarrhoea, abdominal pains and loss of consciousness. Bleeding, paralysis and possible death.

SMALL-EYED SNAKE ★★★★

0.5–1m. Glossy black with pale pink to cream belly. Very small dark eyes. Sometimes mistaken for a small Red-bellied Black Snake but differs in having small eyes and no pink colouration on the lower sides.

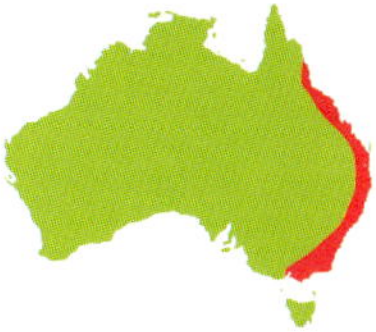

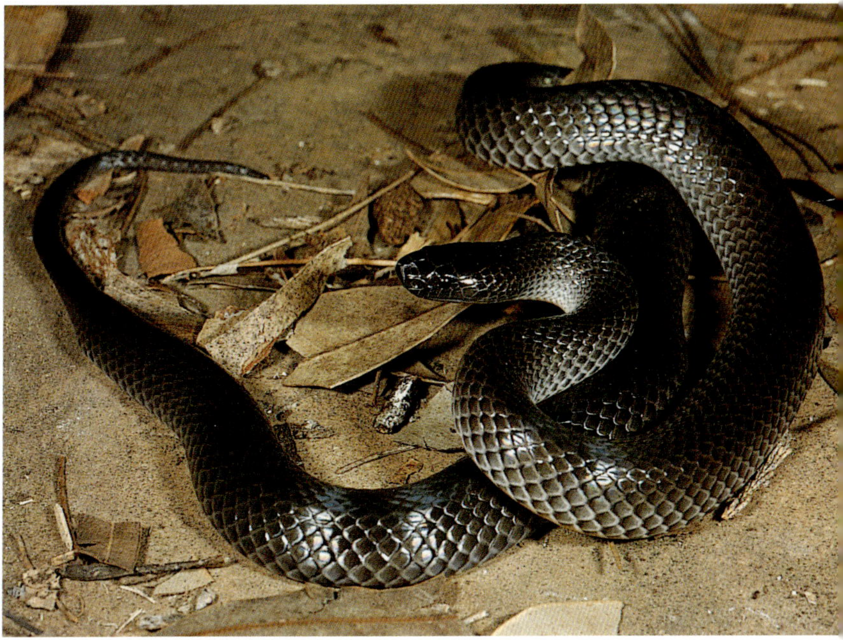

GEOFF SWAN

Symptoms (First Aid — see page 109)

Painful bite. Headache, muscle damage and weakness. One death has been attributed to this snake.

S SPIDERS

SPIDERS ARE more active during the warmer months, and may enter houses looking for a mate or for food. Females generally are larger than males. They can be found almost everywhere and come in many shapes and sizes. All can inflict potentially painful bites, but only the following species are considered to be dangerous. In all cases of spider bite it's useful to collect the spider for positive identification. The safest way to do this is to spray it with insecticide, then put the dead spider in a jar.

REDBACK SPIDER ★★★

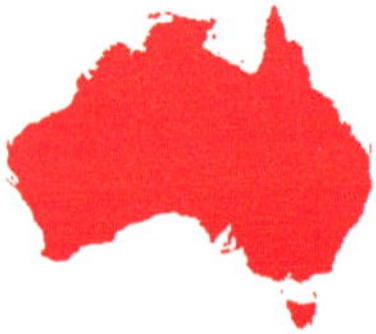

4–14mm long. Female mostly black with a red to orange stripe on top of abdomen. Male much smaller (3–4mm), light brown with or without red stripe. Males and juveniles may have white markings on abdomen. Web is a tangled, tunnel-like structure found in outside toilets, sheds, rubbish piles, letter boxes and among rocks or logs. Usually close to human habitation.

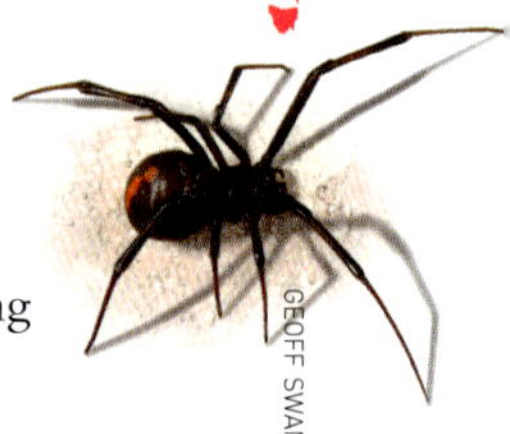

GEOFF SWAN

Symptoms

Bite may be painless, with symptoms occurring several minutes later and increasing in intensity. Common symptoms are pain, nausea and vomiting, sweating (there is always local sweating at the site of the bite) and weakness.

First Aid

- Reassure victim.
- Apply ice pack/cold compress to relieve pain.
- Do not bandage the bite.
- Take analgesics if necessary and seek medical aid.
- Antivenom is available.

BLACK HOUSE SPIDER ★★★

(Window Spider)

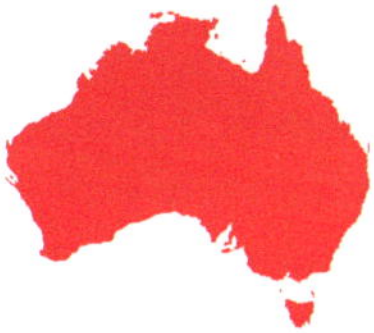

9–18mm long. Robust black spider, with a dark grey abdomen that has whitish flecks. The male is smaller than the female. Web is dense and untidy with a funnel entrance, constructed in corners of window frames, crevices in bricks, fences, tree trunks and similar sites. Sometimes mistaken for a Funnel-web Spider but the two differ in appearance, size and habitat. More common in southern and eastern Australia.

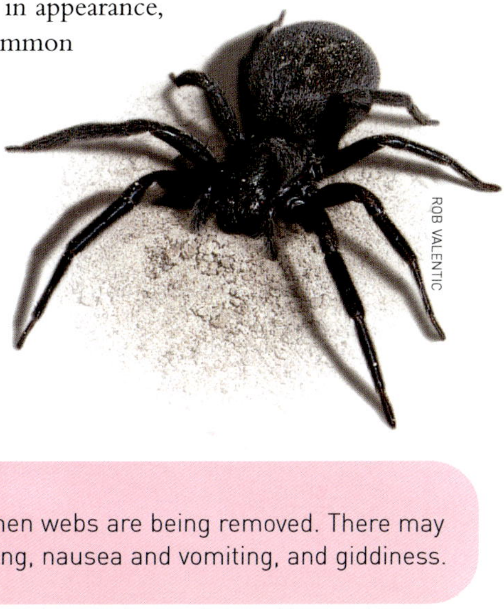

ROB VALENTIC

Symptoms

Bites usually occur when webs are being removed. There may be severe pain, sweating, nausea and vomiting, and giddiness.

First Aid

- Wash the site of the bite.
- Apply ice pack/cold compress to relieve pain.
- Administer an analgesic if necessary.
- Seek medical aid if symptoms persist.

FUNNEL-WEB SPIDERS ★★★★

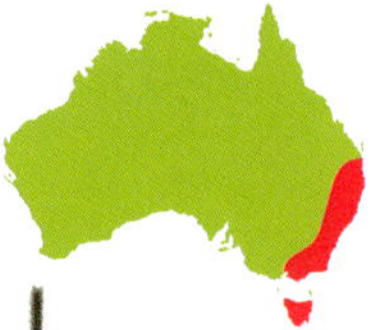

Generally 1.5–4.5cm long. Large, robust spiders with a shiny dark brown to black forebody and a reddish brown to black abdomen. The fangs are large and obvious. Males are smaller and have a spur or projection about half way along the second legs. Both males and females have two obvious projections (spinnerets) at the end of the abdomen. Male is more dangerous than female. Silk-lined burrows are located in moist sheltered spots under rocks, in and under rotting logs, tree crevices and rock piles. Most have irregular silk trip lines radiating out from the entrance. Thirty-six species of funnel-web spider have been identified.

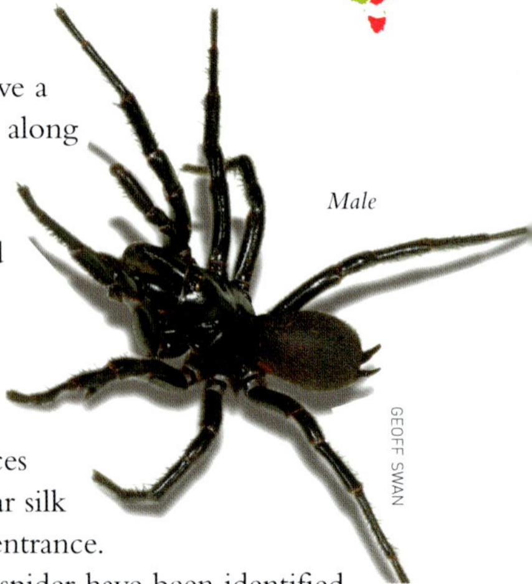

Male

GEOFF SWAN

Symptoms

Local pain, numbness in the mouth, sweating, vomiting, watering eyes, excess saliva, difficulty breathing, coma and possibly death.

First Aid

- Lay victim down and reassure.
- Apply a pressure-immobilisation bandage immediately (see page 15) and splint the bitten limb.
- Seek medical aid urgently.
- Collect spider for positive identification. Antivenom is available.

MOUSE SPIDERS ★★★

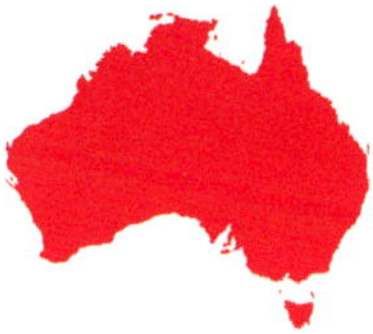

Generally 1–3cm long. Solid, squat spiders with a wide head and very large jaws in proportion to the size of the spider. Males are smaller than females. Females are usually black, but males, depending on the species, can have a red, yellow or orange head and jaws with dark blue, grey, plum red or black abdomen. Dig burrows in the ground. These are silk lined and may have one or two trapdoors. There are several species of mouse spider.

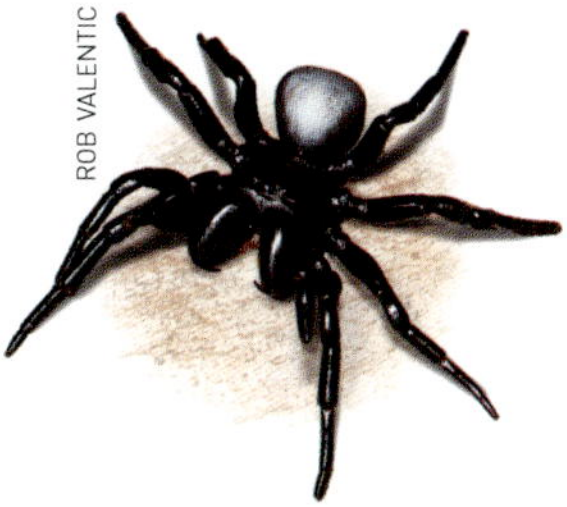

ROB VALENTIC

Male mouse spider

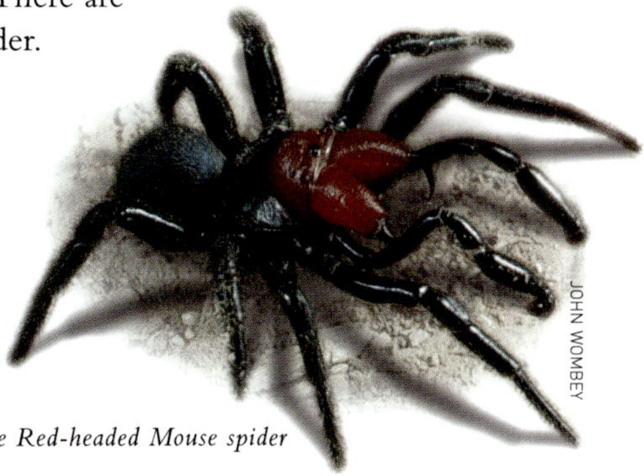

JOHN WOMBEY

Male Red-headed Mouse spider

Symptoms

Very few bites recorded. Local pain and some discomfort. A small child bitten by a male mouse spider went into a coma within 15 minutes.

First Aid

- Lie victim down and reassure.
- Apply pressure-immobilisation bandage (see page 15) and keep victim still.
- Seek medical aid urgently.

WHITE-TAILED SPIDER ★★★

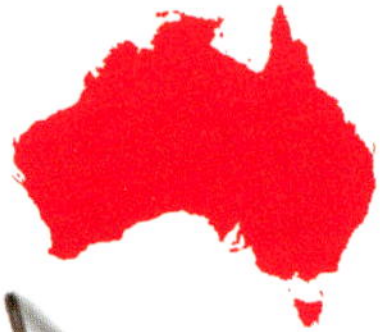

12–20mm long. Dark brown to black cigar-shaped body with a white spot on the end of the abdomen. Preferred food is other spiders and they will often be found in homes hunting house spiders, curtain-web spiders and daddy-long-legs spiders. In the bush under rocks, loose bark and leaf litter.

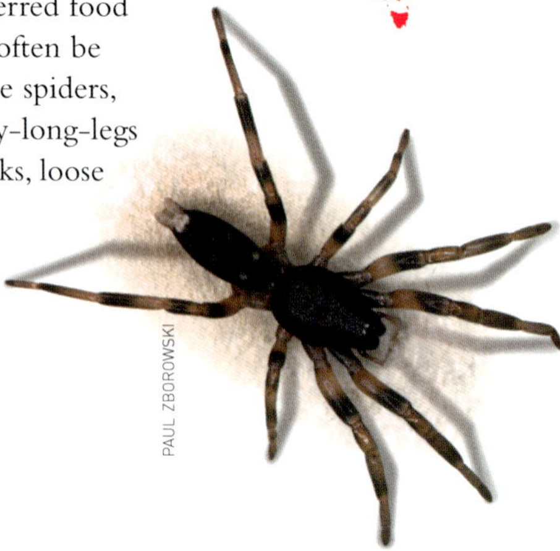

PAUL ZBOROWSKI

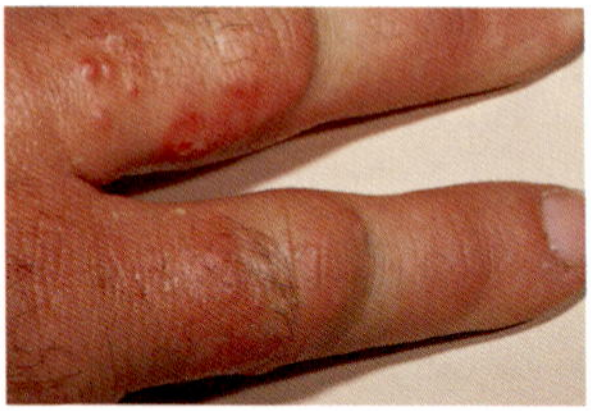

ROB VALENTIC

Bites cause swelling and itching.

Symptoms

An initial burning pain, swelling and itchiness that may last for a few hours or a few days. There has been much anecdotal comment about skin ulcerations following bites by this spider. A study of 100 verified White-tailed Spider bites did not find a single case of ulceration, which suggests that this is an uncommon outcome from a White-tailed Spider bite.

First Aid

- Reassure victim.
- Wash bite with soap and water.
- Apply ice pack/cold compress to reduce pain.
- If any weals or blistering appear, seek medical aid.

SPONGES ★★

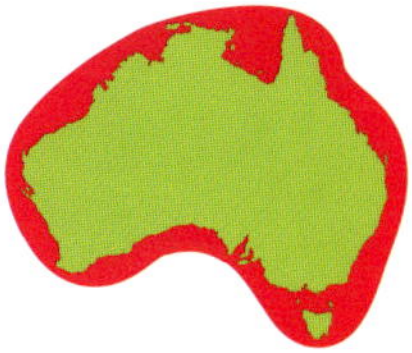

1–5cm. Various colours and shapes. Some are flat and form a crust over rocks. Others cluster together to form tall, bulky growths. Normally live attached to ocean floor where there is constant movement of water from which they filter nutrients.

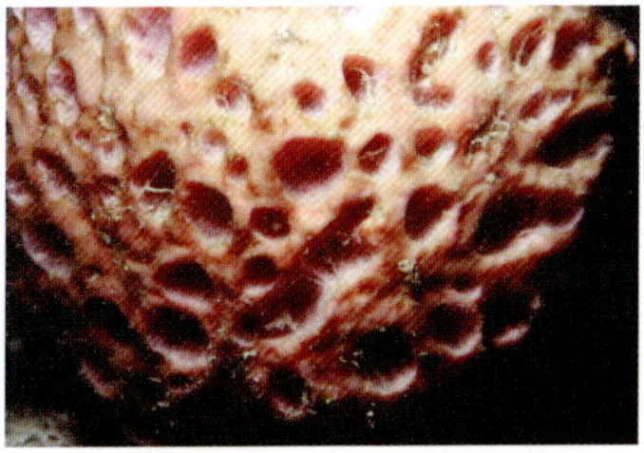

SANDY JACKA

Golf Ball Sponge

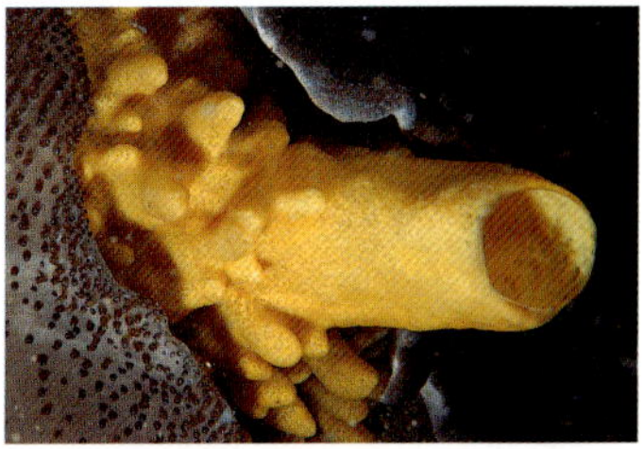

BECCA SAUNDERS

Tube Sponge

Symptoms

Many sponges have very small spikes of silica or calcium carbonate that form part of their skeleton. These are responsible for many of the injuries arising from contact. Some sponges have also developed toxic substances for defence from predators.

A contact dermatitis develops on the skin that has been in contact with the sponge. Irritation may begin any time from five minutes to two hours after contact and can progress to severe itching. Skin may remain sensitive for over a week.

First Aid

- Do not rub the affected area.
- Wash gently with water.
- Apply an ice pack or local anaesthetic cream.
- If symptoms are severe or the victim is distressed, seek medical aid.

S STINGING NETTLE ★

(Scrub Nettle)

20–150cm high. Herbaceous weed with serrated leaves covered in transparent stinging hairs. Both native and introduced stinging nettles occur Australia-wide. Usually found in cooler regions on unused ground, grassland and cultivated land under trees.

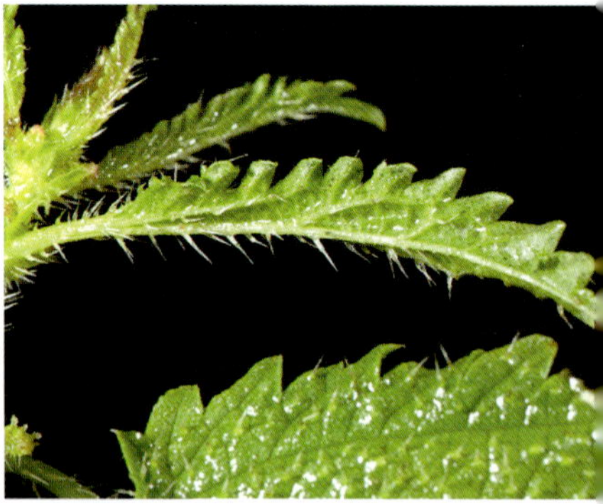

GEOFF SWAN

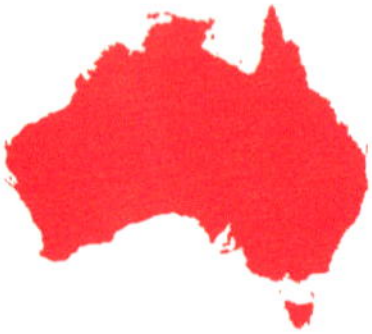

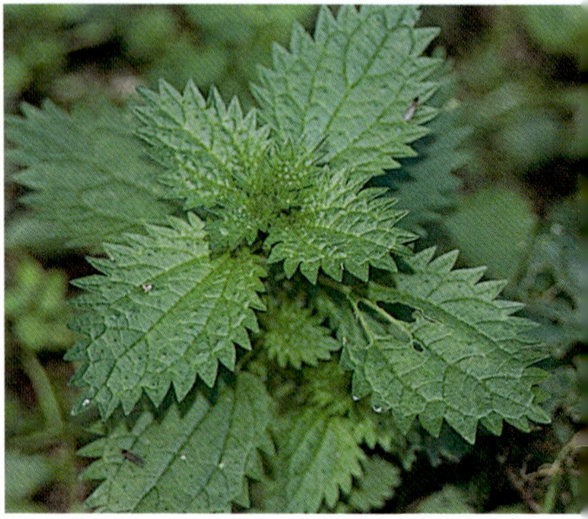

GEOFF SWAN

Symptoms

Irritants in hairs cause a stinging, burning sensation commencing a few seconds after brushing against the leaves. Can leave a rash on sensitive skin and is itchy.

First Aid

- Apply an ice pack/cold compress.

STINGING TREE ★★★

(Gympie, Queensland Stinging Tree, Giant Stinging Tree, Shiny-leaved Stinging Tree, Moonlighter)

2–30m tall. There are several species of stinging tree. Large mulberry-like leaves covered with large stiff hairs. The leaves usually have holes eaten in them due to caterpillar infestations. Clusters of white to pink berries. Restricted to rainforests in NSW and Qld. Occur most frequently at rainforest edges, or where there are clearings or tracks in the rainforest.

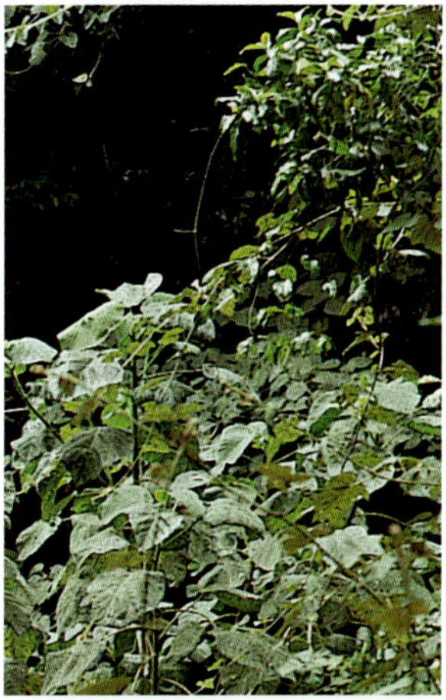

DENISE GREIG

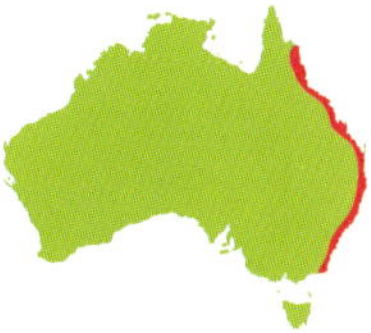

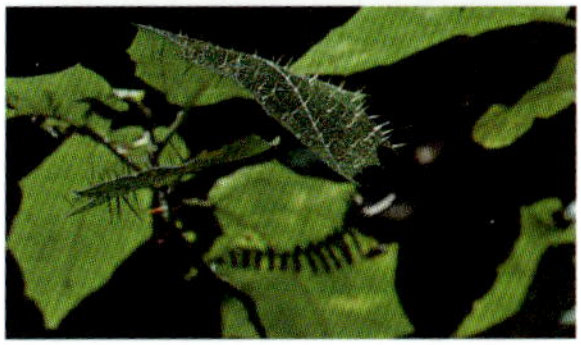

DENISE GREIG

Symptoms

Immediate, severe pain that can last for more than 24 hours. Lymph glands may also become tender and painful. The sting can return weeks or even months later, especially if the area of the sting becomes wet.

First Aid

- Paxyl spray may provide some relief.
- A depilatory wax treatment may help remove the stinging hairs.
- Seek medical aid.

STINGRAYS ★★★

20cm–2.5m wide and up to 4.5m long. Flattened, with a disc-like body and a long, whip-like tail. Sandy grey, silver–green to dark brown in colour, often with spots, stripes or blotches in blue, white or dark brown. At base of tail there are one or more bony spines used for self-defence. Small mouth on underside of body. Side fins or flaps are like large wings. Like sharks, stingrays have a skeleton that is comprised of cartilage, not bone. Coastal and deeper waters. They are curious and will sometimes approach divers. Not dangerous unless stepped upon or molested.

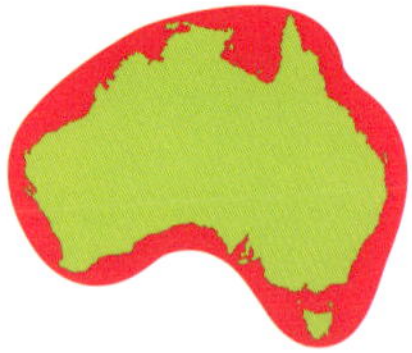

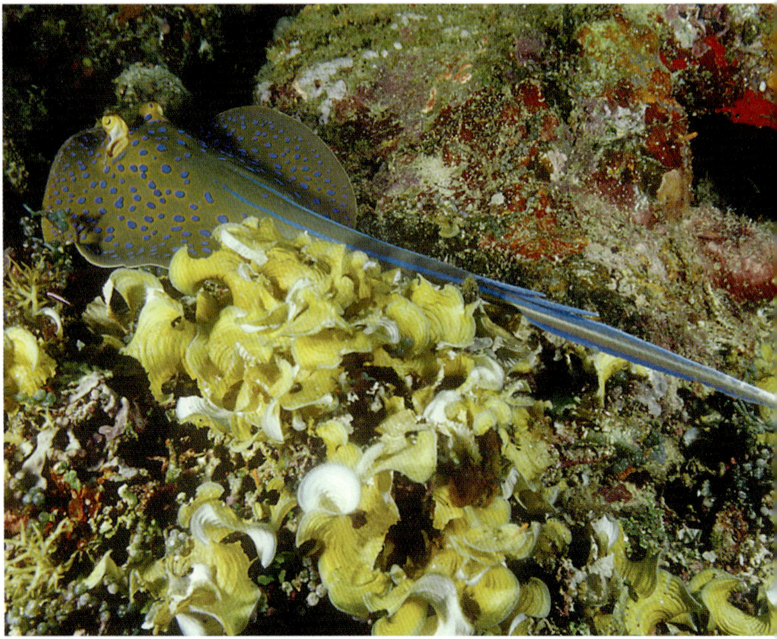

NEIL VINCENT

Blue-spotted Fantail

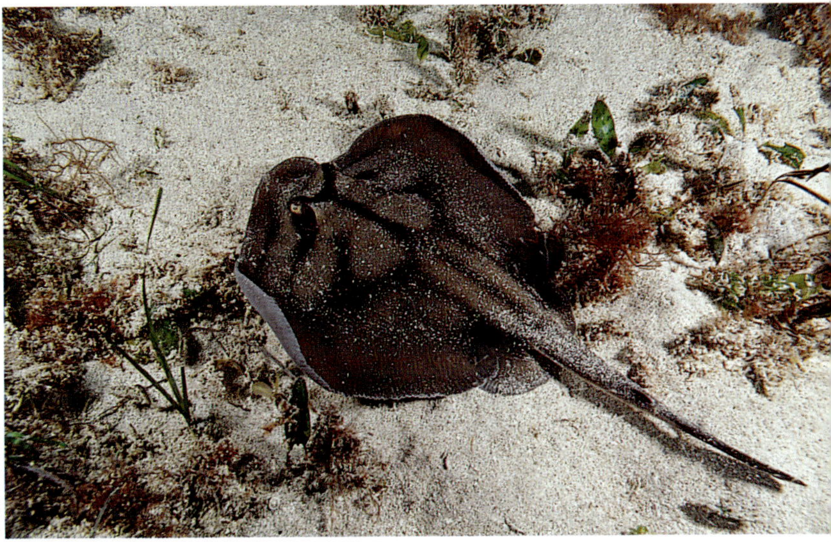

BECCA SAUNDERS

Banded Stingaree

Symptoms

Painful wound inflicted by serrated spine. Wound may be a puncture or laceration and there may be extensive physical damage, depending upon the site.

First Aid

- Remove victim from water and reassure.
- Bleeding can be profuse but may relieve the pain.
- Wash the wound. Hot water can reduce the pain and effects of venom.
- The priority is managing blood loss if the wound is severe (see page 14).
- Seek medical aid.

T TICKS ★★★

0.5–15mm long. Flattened and oval with eight legs. Dark grey to silver–grey to cream in colour. Larval stage has only six legs and is pinhead size. Gorged with blood they resemble a small blood blister. There are many species of tick in Australia and many only feed on a specific animal, such as numbats, echidnas, reptiles or birds. However, a number attack people; the Paralysis Tick is the one that causes the most concern. Ticks will wait in low vegetation and grasp onto a passing victim. They do not drop from trees and they cannot jump. The 'Grass' Tick is the larval stage of the Paralysis Tick.

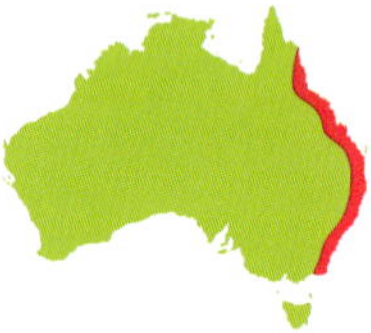

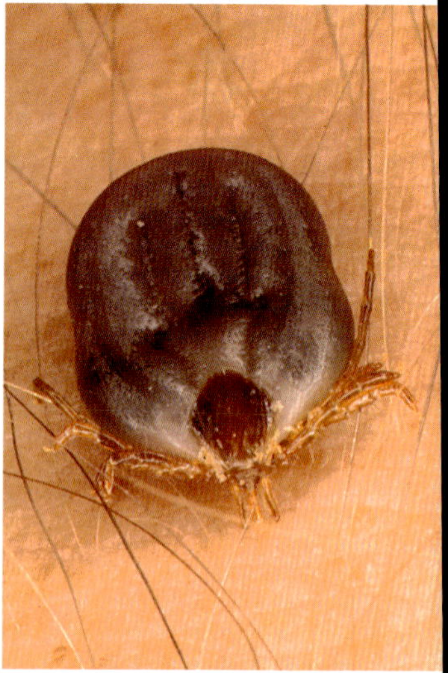

PAUL ZBOROWSKI

Paralysis Tick gorging.

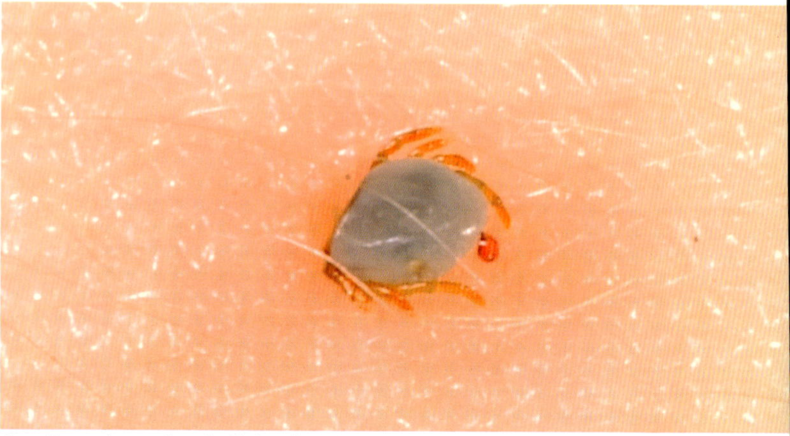

GEOFF SWAN

Juvenile paralysis tick embedded in flesh, feeding.

Symptoms

Itchiness, headache. Bite can cause severe allergic reactions, tick paralysis or tick typhus and may itch for some days after the tick has been removed.

Tick paralysis

Most likely to occur in children. Headache, fever, flu-like symptoms, partial facial paralysis. Develops slowly.

Tick typhus (spotted fever, Flinders Island spotted fever)

Rashes, flu-like symptoms, headaches, fever.

First Aid

- If you've been in a tick-prone area, such as in the bush or in grass, always check out all family members. Ticks may be only pinhead size and can be in the hair, armpits, groin—in fact almost anywhere on the body.
- Kill the tick by applying an insect repellent. Re-apply after a minute or two.
- Wait until the tick is dead (shrivels up), then remove the tick using tweezers. Grasp the tick as close to the skin as possible and pull straight out. Don't squeeze its body.
- If symptoms of tick paralysis or tick typhus develop, or in case of a severe allergic reaction, seek medical aid. A tick antitoxin is available.

W WASPS ★★

MOST OF the wasps found in Australia do not sting people, and are solitary insects. The stinging wasps that people are most likely to come into contact with are the social wasps with communal nests that they will defend vigorously. The native paper wasps and the European wasp are two such groups.

NATIVE PAPER WASPS

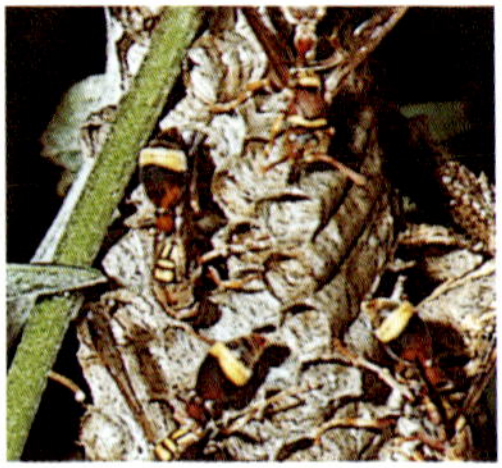

Paper wasp nest

10–15mm long. Usually black and yellow in various combinations, with brownish wings. Small head, very narrow waist. Build paper-like nests under the eaves of houses, in trees or rock overhangs, or underground. Not aggressive unless the nest is brushed against or otherwise disturbed. (If a nest has to be removed, do it at night, spraying with an insect spray.) As their stings do not have barbs, each wasp can sting many times. Bush and suburban areas.

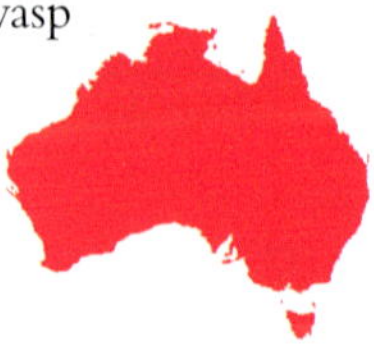

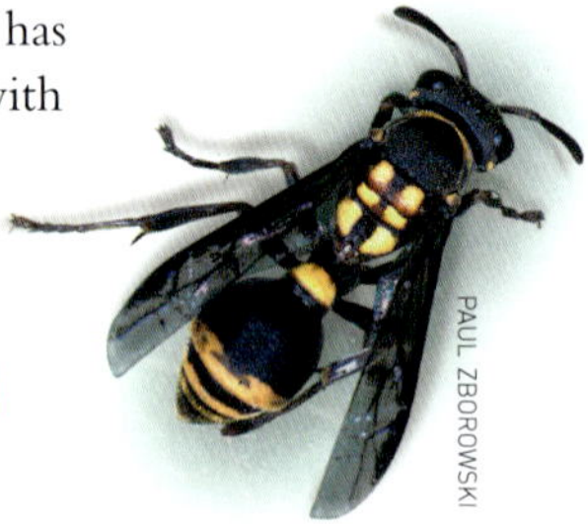

PAUL ZBOROWSKI

Symptoms

A painful sting or often multiple stings.

First Aid

- Move the victim away from the source of the stings.
- Apply ice pack/cold compress to relieve pain.
- If victim is known to be allergic to wasp venom, or if the reaction is severe, seek medical aid urgently.

EUROPEAN WASP

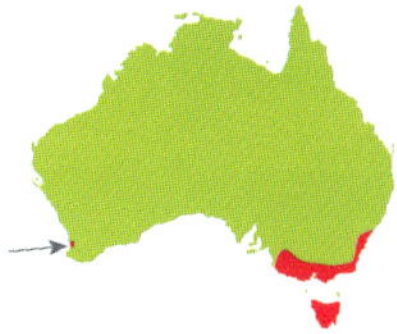

12–15mm long. Stout, with a bright yellow and black banded abdomen.There is a pair of black spots on each yellow band. Clear wings, black antennae. Nest usually underground, in tree hollows, cavities in walls or in ceilings. More aggressive than native wasps or bees and will attack if their nests are disturbed. (Call in professional pest controllers to remove nests.) Attracted to sweet food and drink, and meat, and can cause big problems at picnic areas and barbecues.

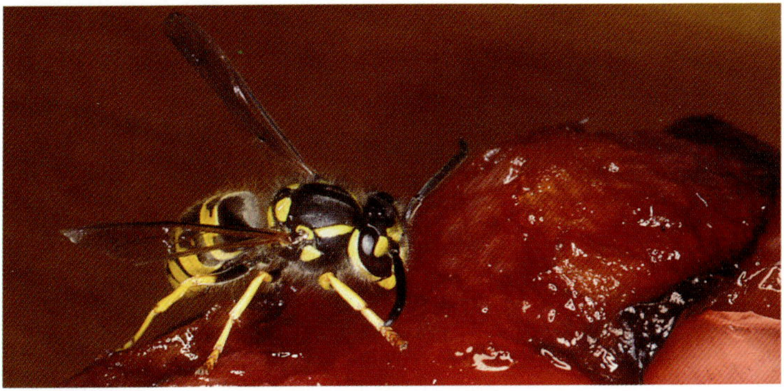

PAUL ZBOROWSKI

Symptoms

The stings cause burning pain and swelling.

First Aid

- Remove victim from source of stings.
- Apply ice pack/cold compress to relieve pain.
- If victim is known to be allergic to wasp venom, or if the reaction is severe, seek medical aid urgently.

WASPS ★★

BLUE ANT

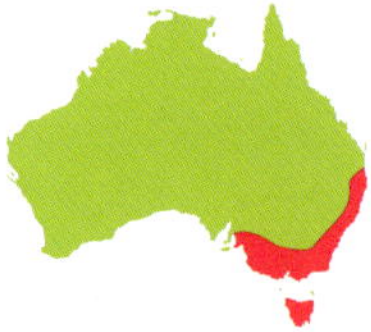

2–3cm long with no wings. These wasps are often mistaken for ants, hence the common name Blue Ant (only applies to female). Female is slender, with a metallic blue body and reddish legs and antennae. She is solitary and hunts on the ground for insect pupae to lay her eggs on. Male is small, black and has wings. Not aggressive but female will sting if molested.

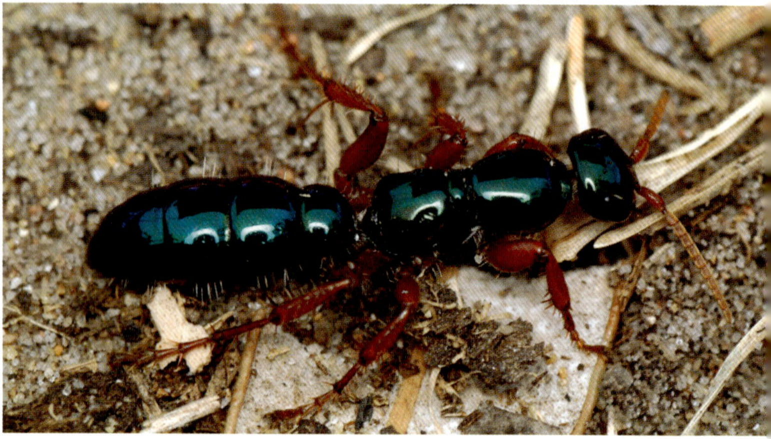

CSIRO

Symptoms

Very painful sting or stings.

First Aid

- Apply an ice pack/cold compress to relieve pain.
- If victim is known to be allergic to wasp venom, or if the reaction is severe, seek immediate medical aid.

INDEX

INDEX